Core Anatomy for Students

Volume 3: The Head and Neck

Christopher Dean

*Department of Anatomy and Developmental Biology,
University College London,
London, UK*

and

John Pegington

*Department of Anatomy and Developmental Biology,
University College London,
London, UK*

WB SAUNDERS COMPANY LIMITED
London   Philadelphia   Toronto   Sydney   Tokyo

W.B. Saunders Company Ltd   24–28 Oval Road
London NW1 7DX, UK

The Curtis Center
Independence Square West
Philadelphia, PA 19106-3399, USA

Harcourt Brace & Company
55 Horner Avenue
Toronto, Ontario M8Z 4X6, Canada

Harcourt Brace & Company, Australia
30–52 Smidmore Street
Marrickville, NSW 2204, Australia

Harcourt Brace & Company, Japan
Ichibancho Central Building, 22-1 Ichibancho
Chiyoda-ku, Tokyo 102, Japan

© 1996 W.B. Saunders Company Ltd

British Library Cataloguing in Publication Data is available

ISBN 0-7020-2042-7

This book is printed on acid-free paper

Typeset by Selwood Systems, Midsomer Norton
Printed in Great Britain by The Bath Press, Avon, UK

Core Anatomy for Students is dedicated to the memory of John Pegington. Few people have thought harder about how to teach anatomy for the first time. Few people have been as successful at it.

Contents

Preface

Core Anatomy for Students was written as a revision text. It was originally intended for students who may have left themselves short of time to work for exams, or for those who may be faced with sitting anatomy exams for a second time. We presume therefore, that students who use one or all of these three volumes will already have completed an anatomy course and will therefore be familiar with basic anatomical terminology. We expect that they will have studied some developmental biology and histology and also that those who use this text will be keen to start their clinical studies and will be curious to know why a good deal of anatomy is clinically important. With these things in mind we have occasionally drawn freely on developmental anatomy and some applied anatomy in each of these three volumes to clarify or to illustrate what we feel is important material.

These volumes are not designed to be used as a standard textbook or reference book of anatomy. They are meant to provide a framework for revision and self-directed learning. They represent a synopsis of basic material that we feel defines a core of useful knowledge. We regard this core as material which lies in the current mainstream of a continuous learning programme such as medicine. It is that which we consider as necessary to know in order to understand the next step in this sequence of learning. The content of each volume is highly selective and many things are deliberately left out. Neither do we intend Core Anatomy for Students to be a set of revision notes where factual details are maximally condensed. Our emphasis here is on a readable text that explains, sometimes at length, what may be difficult or important. On occasions the text is deliberately repetitious. We have tried to promote an understanding of anatomy in a way that reinforces the learning process, which we feel lists of things to be revised and committed to memory do not.

The material presented here is probably not set out in a way that parallels the way it was first taught. We hope that the order in which things are presented makes functional and logical sense and also ties together some topics that may otherwise seem unrelated. Above all, we hope that each section of each volume forms a cogent revision programme in its own right and that dental, medical, speech science, podiatry, physiotherapy and other students who study anatomy find Core Anatomy for Students useful.

Acknowledgements

In the first instance we would like to acknowledge Dr Wojtek Krzemieniewski who drew earlier versions of some of the illustrations we have used. We are especially grateful to Breda O'Connor for typing a great deal of the manuscript and to Dr Deana D'Souza for her scrutiny of the text and illustrations. We are grateful to Barry Johnson and Derek Dudley for technical support and to Jane Pendjiky and Chris Sym for photographic work. In particular, we are grateful to many generations of anatomy, dental, medical, speech science, podiatry and physiotherapy students from The School of Medicine, Ottawa, and from University College London, who have all used earlier versions of this revision text, and who over the years have encouraged us to write more of them, to improve them, correct them and finally to publish them. It goes without saying that the artwork in any anatomy book is fundamental to it success. We are especially grateful to Joanna Cameron for her exceptional illustrations. We would also like to express our thanks to the production team at W.B. Saunders, London.

Introduction

Many people consider the anatomy of the head and neck to be the most difficult region of the body to study. In part, this difficulty arises because complex regions of the head and neck are never understood when they are presented as lists of facts to be learned. In part, much of the difficulty also results from an old-fashioned approach to the subject, the neck, for example, being divided into subregions and triangles that do not follow a functional pattern. All this makes an essentially simple plan difficult to follow.

Volume 3 of *Core Anatomy for Students* is set out in three sections. The first section covers the cranial vault, intracranial region, the eye and the ear. The second section covers the deep neurovascular structures of the neck and the larynx and pharynx. The third section concentrates on the lower facial region, the nose and the mouth.

While each of these sections is complete in its own right and can be studied in any order, we suggest the order they are set out in may be the most appropriate order to work through, since occasional reference is made in later parts of the volume to material discussed in earlier parts.

We have made no attempt to reduce the chapters in each volume to an equal length. As they stand they represent what we feel are coherent functional units which all form part of a sequential revision programme. This means that on some occasions you may have to commit yourself to a fairly lengthy bout of reading. The legends to the diagrams summarize the text and can be used on their own when revising each section on subsequent occasions.

The illustrations are, for the most part, designed to be coloured in as you work through the text. You may choose not to colour any in, or perhaps to colour only certain key diagrams. We would encourage you at least to choose a few key diagrams in each section to colour in, since there is evidence that this helps to commit some of the three-dimensional aspects of anatomy to memory.

At the end of each section there is a revision chapter to help you consolidate your anatomical knowledge and to test your understanding of each region. You may choose to do the multiple choice questions a few at a time as you finish reading each chapter. You may prefer to do them all together at the end of each section. Alternatively, you might even consider doing the even-numbered questions on your first attempt and then the odd-numbered ones on a subsequent occasion. Whatever you decide, remember, they are an integral part of this revision programme and you need to work through them with reference to the text at some stage to get the most out of your learning effort. Do not be tempted to ignore them altogether.

THE INTRACRANIAL REGION, EYE AND EAR

chapter

1

The Skull Vault, Cranial Cavity, and Meninges

The vault bones

The **cranial cavity** contains the brain and meninges as well as all the vessels and nerves that pass to and from the brain. The cranial cavity is surrounded by the **vault bones** at the sides and above, and by the bones of the **cranial base** below. If possible, at this point, you should look at a skull and try to visualize and name each bone that makes up the cranial vault and cranial base. Use Figure 1.1 to guide you.

The bones that make up the vault of the skull are the **frontal, parietal** and **occipital** bones together with a flattened part of the temporal bone, called the **squamous temporal**, and a flattened part of the **sphenoid** bone that is wedged in between the frontal and temporal bones at the side (Fig. 1.1). Interlocking fibrous joints called **sutures** join the individual bones together. The **coronal** suture joins the frontal and the two parietals and this runs in the **coronal plane**. The **sagittal** suture lies between the two parietal bones and runs in the **sagittal plane**. At birth, there is an

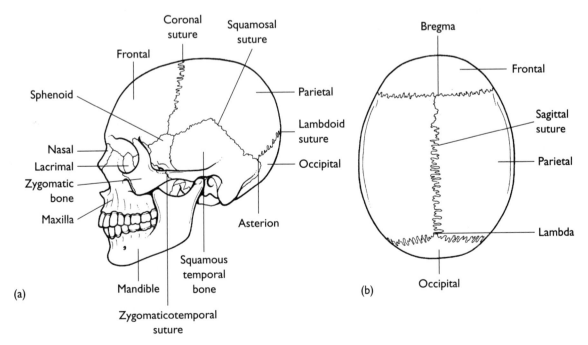

Figure 1.1 Bones and landmarks of the skull seen in lateral view (a) and from above (b).

additional suture in the midline which separates each half of the frontal bone; it usually fuses in the second year of life. This is called the **metopic** suture. The point where the sagittal and parietal sutures meet in the adult is called **bregma**. At birth the bones at bregma are not fully developed and leave a gap which is covered over with fibrous tissue fused to the underlying dura. This is called the **anterior fontanelle** (Fig. 1.2). It may be easily palpated in young babies but it closes as the vault bones coalesce here at around 2 years of age. The point at which the occipital bone meets the parietal bones in the midline is called **lambda**. Seen from the back the **lambdoid suture** looks like the Greek letter λ as it runs inferolaterally on each side towards the mastoid process. (Be sure you understand that there is only one lambdoid suture between the occipital bone and the two parietals, and not one on each side.)

In the neonatal skull (Fig. 1.2) there are more deficiencies between the vault bones both at lambda and at **asterion** and at **pterion**. Asterion is where the temporal, occipital and parietal bones meet; pterion is where the frontal, parietal, temporal and sphenoid bones meet. The bones adjoining the so-called posterior, posterolateral and anterolateral fontanelles (Fig. 1.2) all coalesce and close up these bony deficiencies in the first few months after birth.

In the adult, each bone that forms the vault is constructed like a sandwich, with outer and inner plates or **tables** of compact bone, and with a spongy or trabecular bone called the **diploë** between them (Fig. 1.3). Within the diploë, there is active red blood cell formation (erythopoiesis) throughout life. You will therefore understand why, in some forms of anaemia, the diploë increases in thickness.

The cranial base

The so-called **cranial base** lies beneath the brain (Fig. 1.4). The frontal bones have **orbital processes** that run a short way beneath the frontal lobes of the brain. The sphenoid bone is wedged across the cranial base between the frontal bone and the two temporal bones. The sphenoid bone therefore supports parts of the frontal and temporal lobes of the brain as well as the pituitary gland in the midline. The temporal bones have processes called the **petrous temporal bones** that also run across the cranial base and help to support the temporal lobes of the brain. An obvious feature of the occipital bone is its large foramen, the **foramen magnum**, through which the spinal cord is continuous with the medulla. In front of the foramen magnum the **basioccipital** runs forwards to join with the sphenoid bone. Behind the foramen magnum the occipital bone is cup-shaped and it supports the cerebellum here. Together, each of these parts of

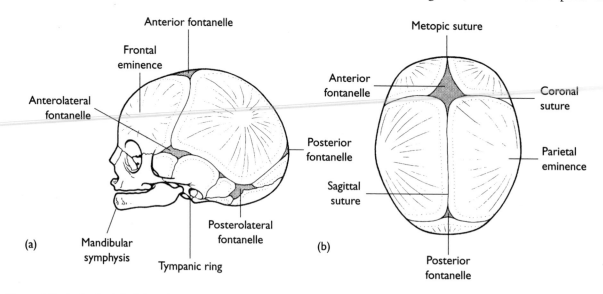

(a) Anterior fontanelle / Frontal eminence / Anterolateral fontanelle / Posterior fontanelle / Mandibular symphysis / Posterolateral fontanelle / Tympanic ring

(b) Metopic suture / Anterior fontanelle / Coronal suture / Parietal eminence / Sagittal suture / Posterior fontanelle

Figure 1.2   In the fetal skull there is no mastoid process and only a ring of bone around the outer margin of the middle ear cavity. A metopic suture divides the frontal bone, and fontanelles extend between the vault bones at various sites. The mandible is also unfused at the symphysis. (a) Lateral view; (b) from above.

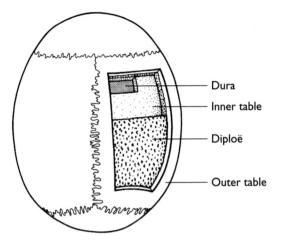

Figure 1.3 Inner and outer tables of cortical bone sandwich a layer of erythropoietic diploic tissue between them.

the frontal, temporal, sphenoid and occipital bones support the brain from beneath. You will notice that the only bones of the vault that do not also contribute to the cranial base are the parietal bones.

The intracranial region

Look now at the interior of the cranial cavity and examine the bones that form its base more closely (Fig. 1.4). The floor can be divided into three fossae called the anterior, middle and posterior **cranial fossae**. The anterior cranial fossa is at a higher level than

the middle cranial fossa, and this in turn is at a higher level than the posterior cranial fossa.

The anterior cranial fossa

Much of the anterior cranial fossa is formed by the two flattened orbital processes of the frontal bone, one on each side. These also form the roof over each orbit. Between the two orbital cavities is a delicate bone whose upper surface only can be seen intracranially. It is called the **ethmoid** bone. The intracranial surface of the ethmoid bone is perforated by tiny holes for branches of the first cranial nerve (I), the olfactory nerve, to run through from the top of the nose. It is therefore known as the **cribriform plate** of the ethmoid bone. In the midline of the anterior cranial fossa, the ethmoid bone is raised into a crest, the **crista galli**. The bone of the ethmoid is frail, like egg shell, and is therefore easily fractured. Injuries to the ethmoid often give rise to a loss of cerebrospinal fluid (CSF) here or bleeding into the orbit (subconjunctival haemorrhage) or bleeding from the nose (epistaxis). The sides of the ethmoid bone are below the level of the anterior cranial fossa and make up the medial walls of both the orbital cavities and the lateral walls of the nasal cavity. The ethmoid bone has a midline septum, called the **perpendicular plate** of the ethmoid. This lies high in the nasal cavity in the plane of the crista galli and is continuous with the midline cartilage of the nose lower down.

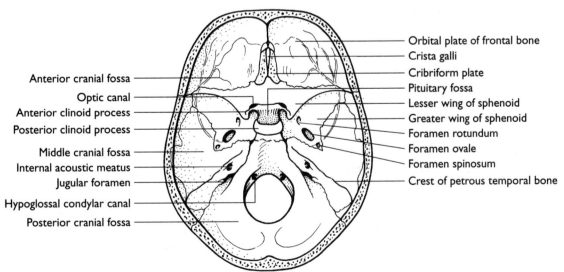

Figure 1.4 The anterior, middle and posterior cranial fossae with important landmarks and foramina seen from above.

Behind the orbital processes of the frontal bone and ethmoid bone in the anterior cranial fossa is a part of the sphenoid bone. The sphenoid bone is complicated and it forms part of both the anterior cranial fossa and the middle cranial fossa. It is composed of a **body** centrally from which **wings** arise and pass laterally. When disarticulated and looked at from the front it is shaped like a butterfly. The wings are four in number but in fact the lower two look more like the legs of this imaginary butterfly rather than extra wings. Look into the orbital cavity of a skull and identify the tear-shaped **superior orbital fissure**. The upper margin of the superior orbital fissure is part of the **lesser wing** of the sphenoid bone, which arises from the top of the body. You will see that the lesser wing also forms the posterior margin of the anterior cranial fossa when you look intracranially. The lower margin of the superior orbital fissure is part of the **greater wing** of the sphenoid bone. This spreads laterally to form the floor and side walls of the middle cranial fossa. It is the flattened outer portion of the greater wing of the sphenoid bone that contributes to the vault at pterion. The superior orbital fissure is always a good place to distinguish between the greater and lesser wings of the sphenoid.

The middle cranial fossa

Turn your attention now to the middle cranial fossa (Fig. 1.4). Much of this is formed by the body and greater wings of the sphenoid bone. Look at the central part of the body of the sphenoid which is raised high in the midline behind the anterior cranial fossa. It presents with a depression in the midline which houses the pituitary gland in life. This is called the **pituitary fossa**, but because of its supposed similarity in shape to a high-backed Turkish saddle it is also often referred to as the **sella turcica**. The pituitary fossa has two **anterior clinoid processes** and two **posterior clinoid processes** at its corners. On each side in front of the pituitary fossa, and in the roots of the anterior clinoid processes, two important passageways in the lesser wing of the sphenoid bone lead through to the orbital cavities. These are the **optic foramina**, which transmit the optic nerves to the eye. Lateral to these, between the greater and lesser wings of the sphenoid bone, you will again see the superior

orbital fissure, but this time from the intracranial side. The superior orbital fissure leads to the orbital cavity. Just beneath it and still close to the body of the sphenoid bone there is a round foramen, the **foramen rotundum,** that leads eventually to the cheek. There are two more important foramina in the floor of the middle cranial fossa. Both of these pass out through the greater wing of the sphenoid bone to the region beneath the cranial base. The most prominent is an oval foramen, the **foramen ovale**, and just lateral to it in a part of the greater wing called the **spine** of the sphenoid is the **foramen spinosum**. The superior orbital fissure, the foramen rotundum and the foramen ovale each transmit a large division of the **trigeminal nerve**, the Vth cranial nerve. The foramen spinosum transmits an artery called the **middle meningeal artery**. This artery creates a deep groove in the bone along its course over the floor of the middle cranial fossa and more so on the inner aspect of the side wall of the cranial vault. The artery is important because, despite its name, it is primarily a nutrient artery to the bones of the cranial vault.

The other bones of the middle cranial fossa are the two temporal bones, left and right. As we have seen, part of the temporal bone is thick and hard, and projects like a pyramid across the middle cranial fossa. The other part is flat and thin, and forms part of the side wall of the middle cranial fossa and cranial vault. The thick portion is called the **petrous** part and the thin portion the squamous part of the temporal bone. The petrous part has a superior margin which forms a thick bony ridge that runs obliquely forwards across the cranial cavity, towards the body of the sphenoid bone. The top edge of the petrous bone is called the **petrous crest** and it forms the boundary between middle and posterior cranial fossae. It is the petrous temporal bone that contains the organs of hearing and balance within its substance.

The posterior cranial fossa

The vertically oriented posterior aspect of the petrous temporal bone forms the anterior part of the posterior cranial fossa. There is a prominent foramen in the posterior aspect of the petrous temporal bone called the **internal acoustic meatus**, which in life transmits the nerves of the organs of hearing and balance as well as a nerve destined to supply the muscles of the face. Further back, the posterior cranial fossa is formed by the occipital bone. A rather irregular hole, the **jugular foramen**, lies between the petrous temporal bone and the occipital bone. It is really a space between two bones rather than a foramen through one. The jugular foramen transmits three important cranial nerves and a large vein, the **internal jugular vein,** which returns blood from the brain to the neck and thorax. However, it is the foramen magnum that dominates the posterior cranial fossa. The spinal cord and medulla are continuous through the foramen magnum but we will see shortly that there are other important structures that pass through it as well. The **hypoglossal canal** runs above the occipital condyle and transmits the hypoglossal nerve, the last (XIIth) cranial nerve, out of the posterior cranial fossa.

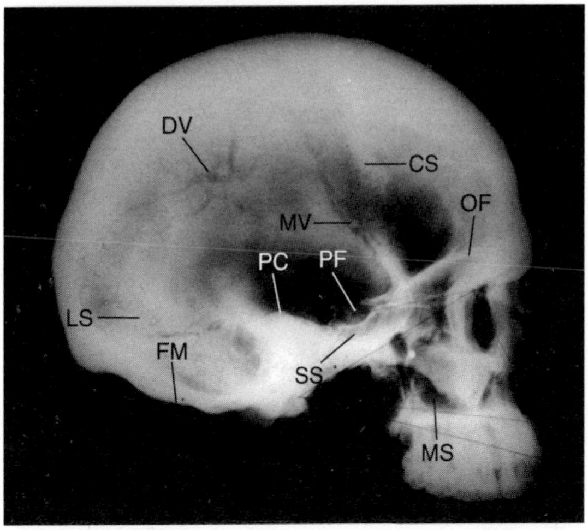

Figure 1.5 Lateral skull radiograph illustrating the orbital process of the frontal bone (OF), the coronal suture (CS), the lambdoid suture (LS), the posterior limit of the foramen magnum (FM), the petrous crest (PC), the pituitary fossa (PF), diploic veins (DV), meningeal vessels (MV), the sphenoidal air sinus (SS) and the maxillary air sinus (MS).

Radiography of the vault bones

Now that we have described the osteology of the cranial fossae it is important to look at one or two radiographs of the skull and identify the bones, sutures and vessels we have mentioned so far. Figures 1.5 and 1.6 illustrate a lateral skull radiograph and an occipitomental skull radiograph respectively. You will notice radiolucent air cavities or **sinuses** in some of the bones around the nose. These bones include the frontal, sphenoid, ethmoid and maxilla. Identify the three cranial fossae and the rounded outline of the pituitary fossa in the lateral skull radiograph. Some of the markings and shadows on the vault bones are formed by blood vessels and others by sutures. Typically there are blood vessels within the diploë (**diploic veins**) that may look like spiders in the parietal region, and these have therefore been called **parietal spiders**. Other vessels, including the middle meningeal artery, make deep grooves on the inside of the cranial vault bones and run across the sphenoid and other vault bones more anteriorly. It is important to recognize the patterns these blood vessels and sutures make on radiographs in order to distinguish them from fractures. Fractures of the skull occur during many head injuries and may involve either the base or vault of the skull. Fractures involving the petrous temporal bone can easily injure the organs of hearing and balance.

The meninges and the cranial venous sinuses

The brain and the spinal cord are covered by three layers of meninges called the **dura mater, arachnoid mater** and **pia mater**. The three layers are continuous through the foramen magnum, the cranial pia being continuous with the spinal pia, the cranial arachnoid with the spinal arachnoid and the cranial dura with the spinal dura.

The cranial dura, unlike the spinal dura, fuses with the periosteum of the internal surface of the vault wherever it is directly in contact with it. This fusion of dura with periosteum takes place over wide areas inside the skull so that when the skull cap is removed the underlying periosteum often strips off the bone as well and remains fused with the outer surface of the dura. The dura itself is a tough collagenous membrane. The middle meningeal artery ascends into the skull through the foramen spinosum and, as mentioned above, although supplying a little blood to the dura, its main function is as a nutrient artery to

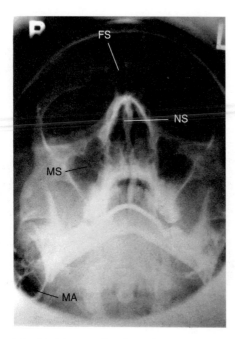

Figure 1.6   Occipitomental radiograph of a patient illustrating the frontal air sinus (FS), the nasal septum (NS), the maxillary air sinus (MS) and the mastoid air cells (MA).

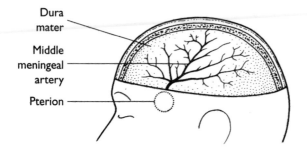

Figure 1.7   The middle meningeal artery enters the cranial cavity through the foramen spinosum and subsequently runs beneath a thin area of vault bone at pterion. The artery runs extradurally and is primarily a nutrient artery to the vault bones.

the bone of the skull. It lies outside the dura and its branches pierce the periosteum to enter the bone (Fig. 1.7). Its course is therefore said to be **extradural**.

Fusion of the dura and the periosteum lining the interior of the skull is, however, incomplete. In places the dura forms folds which pass towards the interior of the cranial cavity in the form of fibrous septa between parts of the brain. In other places long gaps remain between the dura and periosteum in the form of channels, or sinuses, which carry venous blood.

The dura lining the vault of the skull is reflected into the cranial cavity between the two cerebral

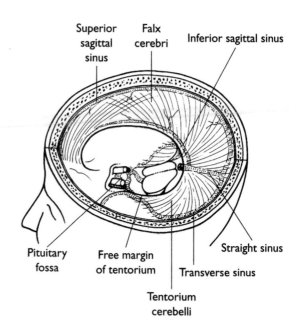

Figure 1.8   The falx cerebri and the tentorium cerebelli partially subdivide the cranial cavity. Cranial venous sinuses run where each of these attach to bone and also between some of the double folds of dura.

hemispheres of the brain as a sickle-shaped fold called the **falx cerebri** (Fig. 1.8). Anteriorly, it is attached to the crista galli, the small crest of bone that projects upwards in the midline from the ethmoid bone in the anterior cranial fossa. At its posterior end the falx spreads into a horizontal fold of dura called the **tentorium cerebelli** (Fig. 1.8). The tentorium cerebelli supports the cerebral hemispheres above and forms a tented roof over the posterior cranial fossa below. The pitch of the tentorium deflects the weight of the cerebral hemispheres out towards the parietal bones, which form the walls of the cranial cavity here. The outer margin of the tentorium runs forwards around the rim of the posterior cranial fossa and on to the crests of the petrous temporal bones and as far as the sides of the pituitary fossa in front. The inner margin of the tentorium is crescentic in shape and free. There is thus a passageway bounded by the body of the sphenoid in front and the free edge or border of the tentorium behind through which the brain stem passes. The brain stem connects the cerebral hemispheres above to the midbrain and pons below. It is worth pointing out at this stage that the inner free borders of the tentorium sweep anteriorly on each side to attach to the anterior clinoid processes. The outer rim of the tentorium which attaches to the

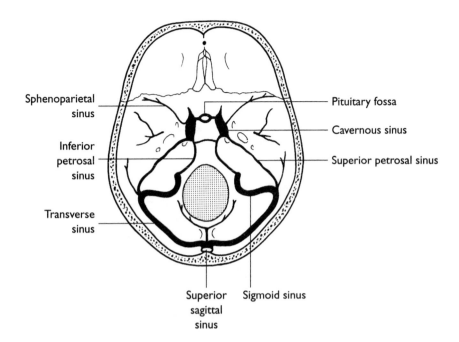

Sphenoparietal sinus

Inferior petrosal sinus

Transverse sinus

Pituitary fossa

Cavernous sinus

Superior petrosal sinus

Superior sagittal sinus

Sigmoid sinus

Figure 1.9 The cranial venous sinuses associated with the floor of the cranial cavity.

petrous crest runs into the petroclinoid ligament anteriorly. This ligament joins the apex of the petrous temporal bone to the posterior clinoid process.

The venous sinuses drain blood from the brain, meninges and skull, mainly into the **internal jugular vein** which leaves the skull through the jugular foramen. We described this foramen already in the posterior cranial fossa. Some of the small venous sinuses, however, are continuous through the foramen magnum with the **vertebral venous plexuses** around the spinal cord. Other venous sinuses also communicate with a number of extracranial veins by means of **emissary veins** which pass all the way through the skull in emissary foramina in the vault bones. **Diploic foramina** transmit diploic veins from the diploë to either the inside or the outside of the vault. They do not then pass all the way through the vault bones like emissary foramina.

The **superior sagittal sinus** is found in the upper border of the falx (Fig. 1.8). It increases in size towards its posterior end. At the point where the falx joins the tentorium, the sinus usually turns to the right to become the right **transverse sinus**. This venous sinus travels around the side of the cranial cavity in the attached margin of the tentorium cerebelli, and then follows an S-shaped curve downwards to the jugular foramen (Fig. 1.9). This latter section is called the **sigmoid sinus**. On passing

through the jugular foramen the sinus becomes the internal jugular vein. As we have seen, most of the venous sinuses occupy slits between dura and periosteum, but two are found entirely between dural folds. These are the **inferior sagittal** and **straight sinuses** (Fig. 1.8). The inferior sagittal sinus is found in the lower free edge of the falx. It joins the **great cerebral vein** from the brain to form the straight sinus. This continues posteriorly to the attached margin of the tentorium to form the left transverse sinus (or occasionally the right).

A **cavernous sinus** is found on each side of the body of the sphenoid bone (Fig. 1.9). These sinuses are very important clinically. Each sinus is large and contains a meshwork of fine fibrous tissue which gives it the consistency of a sponge in life. Several important cranial nerves travel in the dura of the lateral wall of the cavernous sinus on their way to the orbital cavity and to the maxilla or upper jaw. It is easy to remember that the IIIrd and IVth cranial nerves and two divisions of the Vth cranial nerve (Vi, the ophthalmic division, and Vii, the maxillary division) run in the lateral wall of the cavernous sinus (Fig. 1.10). The VIth cranial nerve also runs forwards through the cavernous sinus but is free within the substance of the sinus. It approaches the cavernous sinus from the posterior cranial fossa and passes underneath the petroclinoid ligament to enter it. Within the cavernous

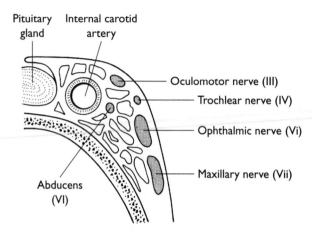

Figure 1.10   The cavernous venous sinus in coronal section. The sinus contains fibrous trabeculae. The abducens and internal carotid artery run through its substance. The oculomotor, trochlear, ophthalmic (Vi) and maxillary (Vii) nerves run in its lateral wall.

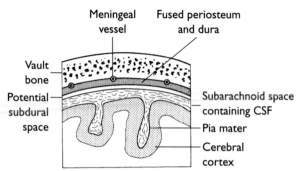

Figure 1.11   Dura mater and periosteum are fused intracranially. Only a potential space exists between the dura and arachnoid but an extensive space, the subarachnoid space, is filled with cerebrospinal fluid (CSF). Pia mater is closely applied to the irregular brain surface.

sinus it travels close to the **internal carotid artery**, which also courses through the cavernous sinus. The VIth nerve also travels to the orbit. We will discuss each of these cranial nerves again when we study the eye and orbit. The internal carotid artery eventually passes out of the cavernous sinus to supply part of the brain with arterial blood.

Each cavernous sinus receives blood from the veins of the orbit. Indeed, it is possible for infections of the orbital cavity or the mid-face to track back through the orbital veins and into the cavernous sinus. The cavernous sinus also communicates with veins below the skull base so that infection from the back of the upper jaw can also track up by this route. Untreated, these may cause thrombosis within the sinus, a very dangerous condition. Each cavernous sinus also communicates with the other across the midline.

Blood is drained from the cavernous sinuses through venous channels which run along the upper and lower borders of the petrous temporal bones. These are therefore known as the **petrosal sinuses**. The superior petrosal sinus occupies the upper edge or crest of the petrous temporal bone. The superior petrosal sinus joins the transverse sinus posteriorly. An inferior petrosal sinus is also found along the lower posterior edge of the petrous bone. It first drains blood from the inner ear by means of a **labyrinthine vein** and then runs to the jugular foramen, where it joins the sigmoid sinus to form the internal jugular vein.

The arachnoid and pia mater

The dura is in contact with the underlying arachnoid but a potential space exists between the two, called the **subdural space** (Fig. 1.11). Many of the veins from the brain drain into the superior sagittal sinus and therefore have to cross this potential space. Rupture of these veins as a result of head injury may give rise to a collection of blood called a **subdural haematoma**. In contrast, rupture of a meningeal artery as described above, perhaps from an injury involving the vault bones, results in an **extradural haematoma** since the artery lies outside or lateral to the dura. We will say more about intracranial bleeds later, in the applied anatomy section.

The arachnoid is a very thin membrane (Fig. 1.11). The outermost part of the arachnoid consists of several layers of flattened cells linked together at their edges by tight junctions to form a continuous sheet. This sheet acts as a barrier to the free passage of ions and molecules into or out of the space between it and the pia mater. The space between the arachnoid and pia is extensive and is called the **subarachnoid space**. This space surrounds the brain and is continuous with that around the spinal cord. It is filled with a clear fluid, the cerebrospinal fluid or CSF.

The pia is a delicate membrane which intimately covers the brain and spinal cord. It dips deeply into the fissures on the brain surface. Blood vessels destined for the brain lie *on the surface* of the pia and anastomose freely. They pierce the pia to enter the brain.

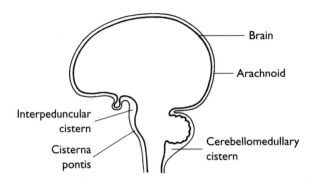

Figure 1.12 Larger subarachnoid spaces, or cisterns, are located in various places beneath the brain.

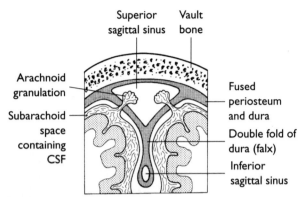

Figure 1.13 Arachnoid granulations are collections of arachnoid villi that protrude into the cranial venous sinuses (especially the superior sagittal sinus). CSF is transported across into the venous circulation at these locations.

Cerebrospinal fluid

Cerebrospinal fluid has both a protective and a regulatory role. It surrounds and buffers the brain and spinal cord against injury and it regulates intracranial pressure, which rises and falls with changes in cerebral blood flow. The fluid is formed inside the cavities or ventricles of the brain, primarily in vascular plexuses. Some of the walls of these cavities are composed only of a thin layer of epithelium and it is here that a vascular network of the pia invaginates it as a series of tufts which project into the cavity. These delicate, vascular tufts make up what are called the **choroid plexuses**. Cerebrospinal fluid is formed as a filtrate leaking from these vascular tufts into the cavities of the brain. The cerebrospinal fluid so formed escapes from the interior of the brain through small holes at the back of the brain stem in the roof of the fourth ventricle and enters the subarachnoid space. From this point it circulates around the brain and spinal cord in the subarachnoid. In certain places the space is large and the cerebrospinal fluid forms pools or **subarachnoid cisterns** (Fig. 1.12). A large lumbar cistern is located at the lower end of the spinal cord and is a useful place to obtain (or tap) cerebrospinal fluid from a patient. Other cisterns are found around the base of the brain.

Absorption of the cerebrospinal fluid takes place through what are called **arachnoid villi**. These are minute protrusions of arachnoid through small openings in the dura forming the superior sagittal sinus (Fig. 1.13). They contain minute tubules which pass through the middle of each villus and which open at the apex into the sinus. When the pressure in the cerebrospinal fluid exceeds that of the venous sinus pressure, the villi fill with cerebrospinal fluid which

then flows into the venous sinus. When the venous pressure increases above cerebrospinal fluid pressure, the villi and their tubules collapse and there is no flow of cerebrospinal fluid. The collections of villi become larger with age and can then be seen with the naked eye on examination of the interior of the superior sagittal sinus. These collections of villi are called **arachnoid granulations**.

If, during an injury to the anterior cranial fossa, the brain coverings in the region of the cribriform plate are torn, cerebrospinal fluid may leak downwards into the nasal cavity (**rhinorrhoea**). If, on the other hand, a fracture of the petrous temporal bone occurs, cerebrospinal fluid may leak through any ensuing cracks into the ear (**otorrhoea**). It is therefore important to ask a patient who has had a head injury whether s/he has noticed blood-stained fluid coming either down the nose or out of the ear.

The blood supply to the brain

Arterial blood to the brain comes from the **vertebral arteries** and from the **internal carotid arteries**. The vertebral arteries are branches of the subclavian arteries in the root of the neck. Each vertebral artery passes into the foramen transversarium of the sixth cervical vertebra (missing out the seventh) and ascends through the series of cervical vertebrae, passing through each successive foramen transversarium. It comes to lie on the side of the lateral mass of the atlas. At this point the vertebral artery winds round

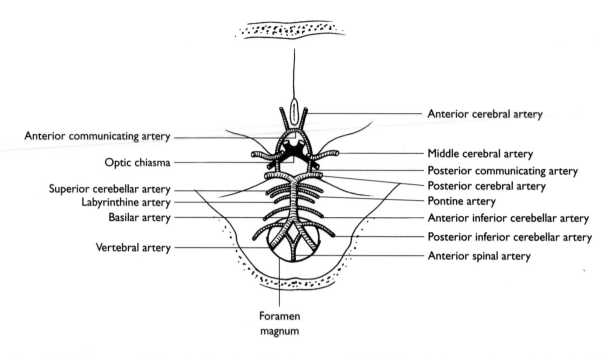

Figure 1.14 The two vertebral arteries join to form the basilar artery, which divides into the two posterior cerebral arteries. Each internal carotid artery divides into an anterior and a middle cerebral artery. Communicating arteries between the the cerebral arteries form a circular arterial anastomosis.

the lateral mass and passes over the posterior arch of the atlas where it enters the foramen magnum. At the foramen magnum it pierces the dura mater and enters the cranial cavity. It runs alongside the lateral aspect of the medulla and then fuses with its fellow of the opposite side in front of the pons to form the **basilar artery** (Fig. 1.14).

The vertebral artery gives off the **anterior** and **posterior spinal arteries** which are extremely important arteries and are pivotal to the blood supply to much of the spinal cord. The basilar artery gives off branches to the cerebellum and to the pons, as well as branches to the labyrinth and inner ear. The basilar artery divides into two **posterior cerebral arteries**, each of which communicates with the **middle cerebral arteries** via the **circle of Willis**. (Just in case you are wondering, Thomas Willis was Physician to King James II and described the circle in 1664.) At the circle of Willis there is communication between all of the arteries that supply the cerebrum. This ensures an equalization of blood pressure and a collateral blood supply should one artery become partially or completely occluded. The posterior cerebral arteries supply much of the occipital and temporal lobes of the cerebral hemispheres.

The internal carotid arteries arise in the neck at

the bifurcation of the common carotid arteries. The internal carotid artery has no branches in the neck (Fig. 1.15). It passes into the carotid canal of the petrous temporal bone and turns a right angle to

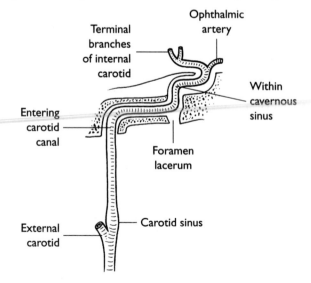

Figure 1.15 The internal carotid artery turns through six right angles as it runs its course through the petrous temporal bone and cavernous sinus. It terminates lateral to the optic chiasma. (After Green JH and Silver PHS (1981) *An Introduction to Human Anatomy.* New York: Oxford Medical Publications.)

travel forwards through the bone to its apex. Here it runs out of its bony canal and across the top of the **foramen lacerum**. The foramen lacerum is simply a cleft between the petrous bone and sphenoid bone that is apparent only in a dried skull since in life it is filled with cartilage. At this point the internal carotid artery turns another right angle to rise into the cavernous sinus, through which it travels forwards. Yet another right-angled turn brings the internal carotid artery up through the roof of the cavernous sinus. Here it lies just medial to the anterior clinoid process. Two further turns, first backwards and then upwards by the side of the **optic chiasma**, brings the internal carotid artery to its termination. Here it divides into the **anterior** and **middle cerebral arteries**. The anterior cerebral artery winds around the genu of the corpus callosum to supply the medial and superolateral aspects of the cerebral hemisphere. The middle cerebral artery enters the lateral cerebral sulcus where it gives off important and delicate branches which supply the internal capsule. It continues on to supply most of the lateral aspects of the cerebral cortex.

One branch of the internal carotid artery is given off just after it emerges through the roof of the cavernous sinus. The **ophthalmic artery** enters the orbit through the optic foramen below and lateral to the optic nerve. It supplies the contents of the orbit and emerges to supply the skin of the forehead and eyebrow. The **central artery of the retina** is by far the most important branch of the ophthalmic artery since this is an end artery and the sole artery to the retina. It runs within the optic nerve to reach the eye. We will discuss the ophthalmic artery later in the context of the orbital contents.

Applied anatomy of the vault and intracranial region

The scalp consists of five layers, the skin and then a dense connective tissue layer beneath, to which the skin is firmly attached; next there is a layer called the **epicranial aponeurosis**, below which is a loose layer of connective tissue; this overlies the deepest layer which is periosteum attached to the bone. 'S C A L P' is the shorthand way of remembering these layers. The epicranial aponeurosis is a tough layer which is attached at the back, the sides and the

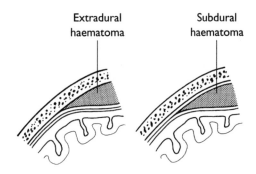

Figure 1.16 An extradural haemorrhage may bleed into a space where the dura and periosteum have stripped away from the vault bones. Subdural bleeds may separate the dura from the arachnoid.

front to the muscles that move the scalp. It is the loose connective tissue layer below this that allows free movement of the scalp.

Normally the dense connective tissue layer beneath the skin forms a sound barrier against superficial infections and lacerations. It is within this dense connective tissue layer that the nerves and blood vessels run upwards and into the skin. Deeper wounds in the scalp do not pull apart if the epicranial aponeurosis is not cut but they do if it is, because the muscles that attach to it pull the aponeurosis in different directions. In this situation the wound gapes and the aponeurosis requires deep suturing.

Blood and infection can track easily in the loose layer of connective tissue beneath the epicranial aponeurosis. There is danger here, because emissary veins may then facilitate communication with the underlying intracranial region and the cranial venous sinuses.

It is important to appreciate the different kinds of intracranial bleeding that can occur. Accidents that involve trauma to the cranium may damage the meningeal arteries and diploic veins within the vault bones. Bleeding is then **extradural** (Fig. 1.16). Prolonged bleeding produces symptoms of compression of the brain. These include, most importantly, increasing drowsiness and eventual loss of consciousnes. Extreme raised intracranial pressure may force the medial part of the temporal lobe of the brain over the free edge of the tentorium cerebelli on the same side as the lesion (Fig. 1.17). This is almost bound to stretch or trap the oculomotor nerve (III). Gradual loss of parasympathetic innervation to the sphincter pupillae muscle results in a pupil that increasingly dilates and will not respond to light.

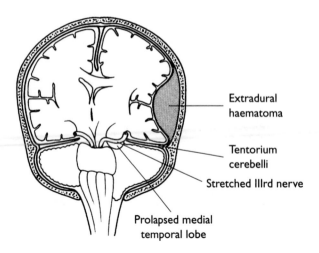

Extradural
haematoma

Tentorium
cerebelli

Stretched IIIrd nerve

Prolapsed medial
temporal lobe

Figure 1.17   Severely raised intracranial pressure may force the medial temporal lobe of the brain over the free edge of the tentorium and in so doing stretch the oculomotor nerve. (After Martin G (1974) *A Manual of Head Injuries in General Surgery.* London: Heinemann.)

Subdural haemorrhage occurs between the dura and the arachnoid (Fig. 1.16) and may, by way of example, follow a blow or box to the head which shakes the brain sufficiently to tear cerebral veins passing from the brain to the cranial venous sinuses. Subdural bleeds may be acute and sudden, or slow and chronic. A slow or chronic subdural bleed may spread and then localize, forming a subdural haematoma or clot. Blood clots can draw in fluid and slowly expand, such that symptoms of a subdural bleed may not begin to appear for up to weeks after the initial accident.

A **subarachnoid** haemorrhage is often sudden and can be mistaken by the patient for a blow to the head. They are very painful because of the immediate meningeal irritation that occurs. A common cause is rupture of a so-called **berry aneurysm.** These are thin-walled outpouchings from the large arteries that supply the brain, which eventually become prone to rupture under continued arterial pressure. This is one cause of what is often called a 'stroke'.

Bleeds into the brain are especially common in old age, more so in people with hypertension (high blood pressure). These are also often referred to as 'strokes'. The middle cerebral artery is a classic site of stroke. Bleeding into the internal capsule of the brain from small frail branches of this artery paralyses the motor nerve fibres travelling from the cerebral cortex to the brain stem and spinal cord. The result is often hemiplegia and loss of speech, which may or may not eventually resolve.

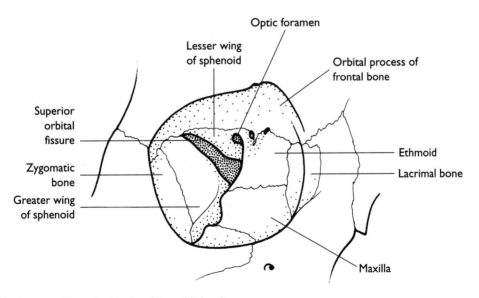

chapter

2

The Orbit and Eye

The orbital cavity

Many bones take part in the formation of the walls and roof of the orbital cavity (Fig. 2.1). Look first at the position of the sphenoid bone. The optic foramen and superior orbital fissure lie within the sphenoid bone. The roof of the orbital cavity is formed by the orbital process of the frontal bone, and on the lateral side the wall is formed by the **zygomatic** bone. In the floor of the orbit the **maxilla** is the dominant bone. A small **lacrimal** bone and part of the ethmoid are found in the medial wall of the orbit and there is even an insignificant contribution from **palatine** bone to the posterior portion of the medial wall of the orbital

cavity. The medial wall lies in the sagittal plane but it is important to realize even now that the lateral wall of the orbital cavity diverges outwards as it is traced forwards.

The eyelids, conjunctiva and lacrimal apparatus

When seen in cross-section (Fig. 2.2) the eyelids consist, from without to within, of skin, a sphincter muscle called the **orbicularis oculi**, the fibrous **tarsal plates** and the **conjunctiva**. There is no subcutaneous

Superior orbital fissure

Zygomatic bone

Greater wing of sphenoid

Lesser wing of sphenoid

Optic foramen

Orbital process of frontal bone

Ethmoid

Lacrimal bone

Maxilla

Figure 2.1 The bones and bony landmarks of the orbital cavity.

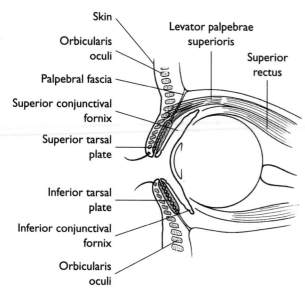

Figure 2.2   Skin, orbicularis oculi and tarsal plates make up the eyelids. The levator palpebrae superioris inserts partially into the top of the upper tarsal plate. It also runs into the fibres of orbicularis oculi.

fat deep to the skin of the eyelids. The eyelashes are found at the edge of the lids; otherwise the skin is almost devoid of hair. The tarsal plates are made of fibrous tissue and they function to stiffen the lids (Fig. 2.3). The inferior tarsus is attached to the lower orbital margin. The superior tarsal plate is larger. Conjunctiva is adherent to their deep surface. Palpebral fascia forms an **orbital septum** which attaches

each of the tarsal plates to the orbital margin. The tendinous fibres of a muscle, **levator palpebrae superioris,** enter the upper eyelid and attach to the upper part of the tarsal plate and also extend beyond this to intermingle with the fibres of orbicularis oculi further anteriorly (Figs 2.4 and 2.5).

The levator palpebrae superioris muscle consists both of voluntary fibres supplied through the IIIrd cranial nerve and involuntary fibres supplied by sympathetic neurons. These fibres together raise the upper eyelid. The **medial** and **lateral palpebral ligaments** connect the margins of the tarsal plates to the sides of the orbit. The medial ligament is strong and lies in front of the **lacrimal sac,** which is the apparatus that collects tears. Two types of glands are found in the lids. The **ciliary glands** are placed immediately behind the roots of the eyelashes. When infected they form a red swelling on the lid margin, called a stye. The other glands are the **tarsal glands.** These are found in vertical rows on the deep surface of the tarsal plates (Fig. 2.4). Their ducts open on to the lid margin. Sensory nerves to the upper lid come from the ophthalmic division of the trigeminal nerve (the Vth cranial nerve), which we will study in more detail shortly, but its branches to this region include the **palpebral branch** of the **lacrimal,** the **supraorbital, supratrochlear** and **infratrochlear** nerves. The **infraorbital nerve** is a branch of the maxillary division of the trigeminal nerve and its branches supply the lower lid.

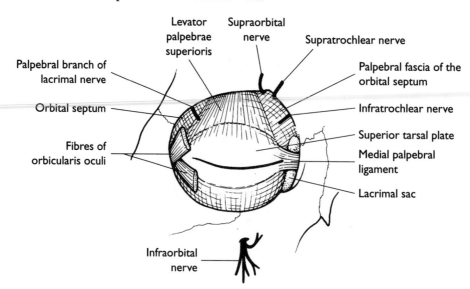

Figure 2.3   Palpebral fascia attaches the tarsal plates to the bone of the orbital margin. The medial and lateral palpebral ligaments anchor the tarsal plates to the sides of the orbital margin.

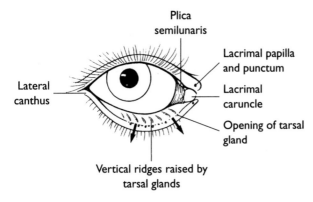

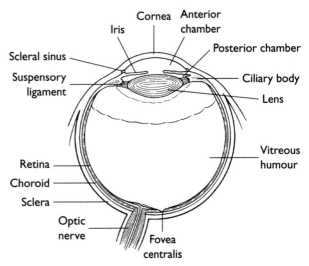

Figure 2.4 Tarsal glands open along the margin of the eyelid. The lacrimal puncta are located on the lacrimal papillae in the medial canthus. The plica semilunaris and the lacrimal caruncle are also found in the medial canthus of the eye.

The orbicularis oculi is a large muscle that surrounds the eye and which consists of several parts. The orbital part is large and wide. Its fibres arise from the medial palpebral ligament and surrounding bone, and sweep around the forehead, temple and cheek to return to this medial point of origin. The palpebral part is smaller. It also arises from the medial palpebral ligament, and loops around the eye. However, it is found entirely within the eyelids. There is also a small lacrimal part which arises from bone behind the lacrimal sac and passes laterally into the eyelids. This part of the orbicularis oculi therefore runs behind the lacrimal apparatus; its function will become clear when we study the lacrimal apparatus in more detail.

Conjunctiva lines the deep surface of the eyelids and the exposed surface of the eye. It is continuous with the anterior epithelium of the cornea. Above and below, where the palpebral parts are reflected on to the eyeball, the recesses are called the **fornices**. The conjunctiva is kept moist at all times. The elliptical space between the two lids is called the **palpebral fissure**. At its extremities this fissure is named the medial and lateral **canthus**. A small red mass, the **lacrimal caruncle**, and a semilunar fold, the **plica semilunaris**, (all that remains of the third eyelid) both lie in the medial canthus.

The lacrimal gland lies mainly in the orbit. However, it does have a small palpebral part which extends into the upper lid. About 12 or so ducts from the gland open into the upper fornix. Lacrimal fluid is produced by the gland and flows towards the medial angle of the conjunctival sac. Within the medial end of each eyelid is a small duct called the **lacrimal canaliculus** (Fig. 2.4). The opening of each of these

Figure 2.5 Structures of the eye seen in horizontal section.

ducts is visible on examination of the eye and is called a **lacrimal punctum**. The punctum opens at a swelling or **lacrimal papilla**, on the medial end of each lid margin. Tears are drawn through the lacrimal canaliculi and into the **lacrimal sac**. This sac lies in a cavity in the medial wall of the bony orbit. From here tears drain downwards through the **nasolacrimal duct** and then into the cavity of the nose. Secretion of the lacrimal gland is initiated by parasympathetic fibres. These follow a devious route to reach the gland and we will study their course later.

Because the attachment of the lacrimal part of the orbicularis oculi and the palpebral part lie either side of the lacrimal sac on the medial side of the orbit, contraction of this muscle squeezes the lacrimal sac. Tears are drawn into the sac as the muscle relaxes. From here they pass into the nasolacrimal duct, which opens into the lateral wall of the nose. The palpebral part of orbicularis oculi is responsible for gently closing the eyes during sleep and when blinking. The orbital part that extends beyond the eyelids screws up the eyes to provide added protection.

The eyeball

The wall of the eye is composed of three coats, the **sclera**, **choroid** and **retina**. The outer of these is transparent in front and is called the **cornea**; behind it is dense and white (Fig. 2.5). The cornea is continuous with the conjunctiva at its margin. There is a layer of epithelium on the front of the cornea and a so-called **posterior limiting lamina** on its posterior surface, which is elastic. At its periphery, around the posterior margin of the cornea, the posterior limiting lamina breaks up into bundles with tiny spaces between them and becomes a permeable structure called the **pectinate ligament** of the iris. These spaces allow **aqueous humour** from the anterior chamber of the eye to pass into a venous sinus in the sclera. It is the means by which aqueous humour is filtered back into the venous system. (This is another example of special body fluids re-entering the venous system. Think once again of lymph and CSF.) Blockage in this system produces a marked increase in fluid pressure in the eye, with damage to sight. The condition is called **glaucoma**.

The sclera is dense and the optic nerve enters through it about 3 mm to the nasal side of the posterior pole. At this point the optic nerve is still surrounded by all three layers of meninges. These fuse with the sclera and the nerves pass through holes in the sclera together with blood vessels. Short and long ciliary nerves and blood vessels also pierce the sclera.

The middle coat of the eye is formed by the iris in front and the choroid behind. The **ciliary body** lies between the two. The ciliary body has the iris attached to its anterior surface and the lens attached to its inner **ciliary process**. Its outer part is composed of the **ciliary muscle**. The iris lies near the front of the eye with the cornea anterior to it and the lens posterior. The cavity between cornea and iris is called the **anterior chamber** of the eye; that between the iris and lens is the **posterior chamber**. Both are continuous through the aperture of the iris and both contain watery aqueous humour. Aqueous humour is formed in the anterior portion of the ciliary process in the posterior chamber of the eye and is then filtred off into the venous sinus of the sclera via the anterior chamber of the eye. The posterior part of the ciliary process is raised into radial ridges by the **suspensory ligament of the lens**, which attaches to it here.

The periphery of the iris is connected to the pectinate ligament and also to anterior part of the ciliary body. The iris contains pigment, which gives it colour. The aperture of the iris is called the pupil and it varies in size according to the light conditions in the surrounding environment. In a dark room the pupil will be widely dilated whereas in bright sunlight it will be constricted. Sympathetic impulses dilate the pupil and parasympathetic impulses constrict it. The diameter of the pupil is governed by muscle fibres in the iris. The **sphincter pupillae** consists of circular fibres arranged around the pupillary margin of the iris (Fig. 2.6). The muscle is activated by parasympathetic fibres which enter the eye through the short ciliary nerves. The **dilator pupillae** is composed of muscle fibres which radiate outwards from the pupillary margin of the iris. They are supplied by sympathetic neurons, most of which arrive in the long ciliary branches of the nasociliary nerve.

The **ciliary muscle** lies within the ciliary body and on microscopic examination can also be seen to have radiating (or meridional) fibres and circular muscle fibres. The radiating fibres arise from the **scleral spur** close to the point at which the sclera and the cornea join. These fibres radiate back into the ciliary process (Fig. 2.6). The circular muscle fibres of the ciliary muscle form a muscular ring near the periphery of the iris. The ciliary muscle is supplied by parasympathetic fibres. When the eye is looking at a distance the lens is fairly flat in shape. In this situation the suspensory ligament pulls on the periphery of the lens to maintain this flattened shape. Contraction of the ciliary muscle both draws the suspensory mechanism of the lens forwards and reduces the diameter of the rim to which the suspensory ligament is attached. This relaxes the peripheral pull of the suspensory ligament on the lens (Fig. 2.7). The lens then takes up its natural resting fat shape. The lens assumes this thick, fat state when looking at an object at close quarters. Contraction of the ciliary muscle therefore occurs when there is a shift from long to short vision. It is a way of focusing on near objects. At the same time there is also constriction of the pupil (both parasympathetic effects, you will note). The eyes also converge when close objects are observed. **Accommodation,** as it is known, consists therefore of several complicated reflexes.

The choroid is the largest part of the middle coat and contains many blood vessels. The inner layer of the eye is the retina. The histology of the retina is important in an understanding of the function of the eye. The retina may be studied in patients by means of an ophthalmoscope. The whole view of the back of the retina seen in this way is called the **fundus**. With this instrument three things can be seen, the **optic disc**, the **macula lutea** and the **retinal arteries** and **veins** (Fig. 2.8). The optic disc is found 3 mm to the nasal side of the anteroposterior axis of the eye. It is

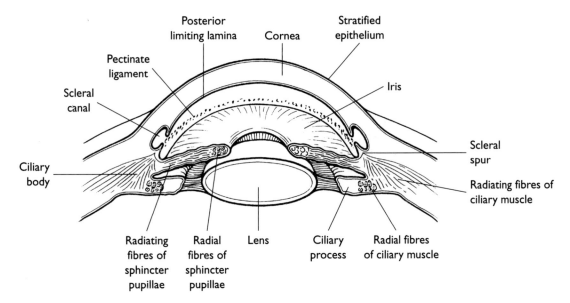

Figure 2.6 Aqueous humour is produced by epithelium on the anterior part of the ciliary process in the posterior chamber. The suspensory ligament of the lens also arises from the ciliary process. Small perforations of the pectinate ligament allow aqueous humour to filter into the venous sinus of the scleral canal. The iris contains circular muscle fibres (sphincter pupillae) and radiating muscle fibres (dilator pupillae). (After MacKinnon P and Morris J (1990) *Oxford Textbook of Functional Anatomy*, Vol. 3. Oxford: Oxford University Press.)

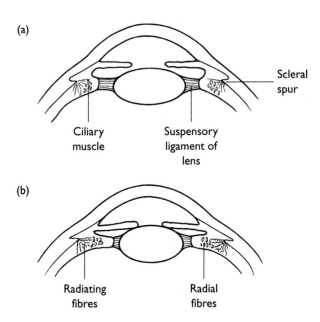

Figure 2.7 The ciliary muscle, part of the ciliary body, arises both as radiating fibres from the scleral spur, which when they contract draw the ciliary body forwards, and as circular muscle fibres, which when they contract reduce the diameter of the rim of the ciliary process to which the suspensory ligament of the lens attaches. Contraction of the ciliary muscle fibres relaxes the pull of the suspensory ligament and allows the lens to assume its natural rounded shape.

where the optic nerve fibres and blood vessels leave the eye. The fibres build up into a circular zone as they leave. This gives the disc a 'raised edge'. The central part of the disc is depressed. The central artery of the retina enters at the disc and its branches can easily be seen here. Retinal veins are also clearly visible.

Lying exactly in the visual axis is a small yellowish spot called the **macula**, the area of most distinct vision. In its centre is a small depression, the **fovea centralis**. At this point the resolving power of the retina is maximal and it is, therefore, the point of most accurate central vision. Increase in intracranial

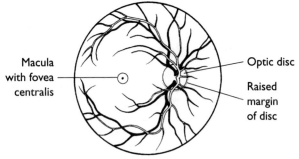

Figure 2.8 The fundus of the eye (the field of view seen through an ophthalmoscope) includes the optic disc with its raised margin, the macula and central fovea, as well as veins (wider vessels) and arteries (narrower vessels) of the retina.

pressure causes the margins of the optic disc to become swollen. This is a useful sign for recognizing and monitoring the progress of certain conditions. The state of the retinal vessels is extremely important to note. It is the one place in the body where vessels may be viewed directly. In patients with high blood pressure the vessels will often have thick walls and appear rigid. Where arteries cross veins they will compress them. Sometimes there will be haemorrhage into the retina from the vessels or white fluffy areas of exudate from vessels. Other conditions such as diabetes also give characteristic appearances when the fundus is examined.

The cavity behind the lens (Fig. 2.5) contains the **vitreous humour**. This is like jelly. In front, the posterior surface of the lens and the ciliary processes form a concavity in the jelly. This is called the **hyaloid fossa**. A minute canal runs from the optic disc to the posterior surface of the lens, called the **hyaloid canal**. It represents the remains of a small branch of the central artery of the retina that degenerates before birth, and can be seen only with special optical instruments. The vitreous body is condensed superficially to form an envelope called the **vitreous membrane**. This is thickened in front to form the **capillary zonule**. While the posterior layer of this is very thin, the anterior layer is thick and forms the suspensory ligament of the lens (Fig. 2.7). It is this ligament that holds the lens in the hyaloid fossa and maintains tension on the periphery of the lens when the eye is at rest or focused on distant objects. Remember that when the ciliary muscle contracts it pulls the ciliary processes, the zonule and suspensory ligaments forwards. This releases tension in the ligaments. The lens then takes up a fat shape by its own elasticity, and its focal length is shortened.

The extraocular structures

The eyeball lies in the orbit surrounded by a fascial sheath (Fig. 2.9) in which it rotates and which separates it from the orbital muscles and fat. The diameter of the eyeball is about 2.5 cm but the cornea is much more curved than the globe. The fascial sheath is deficient in front over the cornea. Posteriorly, the sheath fuses with the dura over the optic nerve. As each extraocular muscle passes to the eyeball it has to pierce the sheath before it can insert into the sclera.

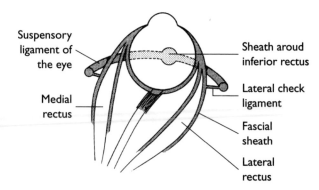

Figure 2.9 Fascial sheaths that extend along the extraocular muscles are fused to the suspensory ligament of the eye by medial and lateral check ligaments. These suspend the eye between the zygomatic bone and the medial wall of the orbital cavity.

It does this close to the equator of the eye, and the sheath is carried on over the muscle here for a short distance. At this point the sleeves of the medial and lateral rectus muscles are attached to the walls of the bony orbit by small fascial slings or **check ligaments**. These help to stabilize the eye in the orbital cavity. They also resist compression of the globe of the eye when the muscles act. The **suspensory ligament** is a hammock-shaped band stretched between the lacrimal and zygomatic bones. It is also attached to the fascial sheath of the eyeball since it blends with the sheaths covering the extraocular muscles that lie beneath the eye.

A **tendinous ring** surrounds the apex of the orbit and encloses the optic foramen and the medial part of the superior orbital fissure (Fig. 2.10). Four muscles

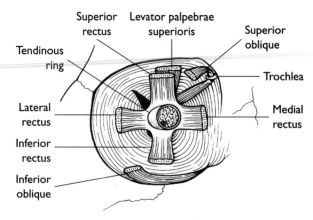

Figure 2.10 Four extraocular muscles arise from a tendinous ring that surrounds both the optic nerve and ophthalmic artery as well as the medial part of the superior orbital fissure. Other extraocular muscles arise from the bone of the orbital cavity.

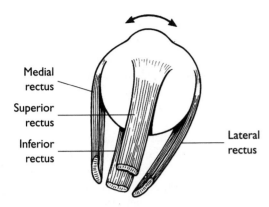

Figure 2.11   The medial and lateral rectus muscles adduct and abduct the eye in the horizontal plane.

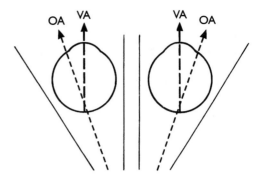

Figure 2.12   When both eyes look directly forwards the visual axis does not correspond to the orbital axis.

arise from this ring and pass forwards to insert in front of the coronal equator of the globe of the eye. These muscles are the **lateral**, **medial**, **superior** and **inferior rectus** muscles. As they pass forwards from their origins they therefore form a cone of muscles around the eye. Two **oblique muscles** arise from the bony orbit outside the cone, one above and one below. The superior oblique muscle arises from bone above the tendinous ring and passes forwards along the upper border of the medial rectus to reach a fibrous pulley, or **trochlea**, attached to the roof of the bony orbit. As the tendon of the muscle passes through this pulley it changes course and is then directed posteriorly to its insertion *behind the coronal equator* of the eye. The inferior oblique muscle arises well forward on the orbital floor, and runs back to insert into the eye *behind* the coronal equator. The levator palpebrae superioris arises from the bony orbit above the origin of the superior rectus and, as we have seen, passes forwards to insert into the structures of the upper eyelid. Its action is to raise the upper eyelid.

It is easy to understand how the lateral and medial recti rotate the eye around a vertical axis through the globe, so that the cornea points laterally and medially respectively (Fig. 2.11). However, the functions of superior and inferior recti need a little more thought. The visual axis lies in the sagittal plane when we look directly forwards at a distant object. Recall that this is parallel with the medial wall of the orbit but not with the lateral wall (Fig. 2.12). Only when the eye is turned *laterally* does the visual axis correspond with the line of pull of the superior and inferior recti. It is therefore only with the eye in this position that their pull is powerfully and directly up and down (Fig. 2.13).

On the other hand, when the eye looks *medially*, the pull of the superior and inferior recti are ineffectual in elevation and depression, and have a tendency to rotate the globe only around a transverse anteroposterior axis. This is called torsion (Fig. 2.14). It is the obliques that become the powerful depressors and elevators in this eye position. Remember that the insertion of each oblique muscle is *behind* the equator of the globe, so that the superior oblique pulls the eye down and the inferior oblique muscle up when the

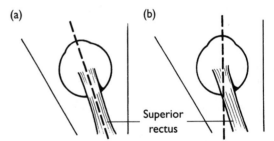

Figure 2.13   When the eye looks laterally, and the orbital and visual axes correspond, the superior and inferior rectus muscles are then also aligned along the visual axis and are perfectly positioned to pull the eye directly up and down.

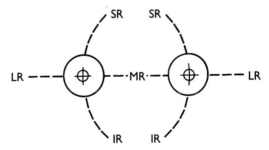

Figure 2.14   Because the direction of pull of the superior and inferior rectus muscles lies in the orbital axis and not in the visual axis when a subject looks directly forwards (Fig. 2.13b), they tend also to draw the eye inwards as the eye is moved up and down.

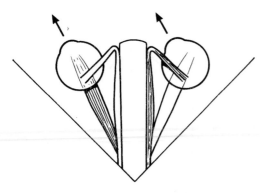

Figure 2.15 When the eye looks medially towards the nose, the pull of the superior oblique muscle is aligned with the visual axis and perfectly positioned to pull the eye directly down. When the eye looks laterally, however, the pull of the superior oblique muscle is across the equator of the eyeball such that it can only roll, or intort, the eye on its central axis.

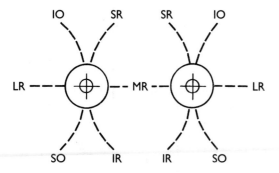

Figure 2.16 When looking directly forwards the combined pull of the obliques and the superior and inferior recti together move the eye directly up and down. To separate the actions of these muscles the eye must be placed in a medial or lateral gaze and the subject asked to follow an object up and down in each position. The lateral and medial recti move the eye from side to side.

eye looks medially. Their actions of elevation and depression are maximally effective when the eye is directed medially (Fig. 2.15). With a laterally directed eye, the obliques become muscles of torsion and have a tendency to rotate the globe only around a transverse anteroposterior axis.

If you examine the eye of a patient who is looking directly at you, asking him or her to look towards his or her nose and then away from it will test the functions of the medial and lateral recti of the eye. Asking the patient to look directly forwards and then up and down will test the obliques together with the superior and inferior recti, but each muscle action cannot be isolated by this method of examination (Fig. 2.16). It is, however, possible to test the individual actions of the obliques and the superior and

inferior recti by first putting the eye into a medial or lateral gaze and then testing elevation and depression. With the eye looking medially it is the *obliques* that are the muscles most suited to elevate and depress (Fig. 2.15). With the eye looking laterally it is the superior and inferior recti that are most suited to be elevators and depressors.

To keep the eyes parallel at all times involves very fine control of the muscles of both eyes. Not only are the pure movements of elevation, depression, lateral and medial motion important but there must be constant corrections for torsional movements.

Neurovascular structures within the orbit

Neurovascular structures enter and leave the orbit through either the optic foramen or the superior orbital fissure. Structures passing through the optic foramen and the medial end of the superior orbital fissure enter the orbit *within* the cone of muscles. Those passing through the lateral part of the fissure must lie *outside* the cone of muscles.

Once the bony roof of the orbit has been removed, three nerves can be seen lying just deep to the periosteum. These enter the orbit through the lateral part of the fissure and lie outside the cone of muscles (Fig. 2.17). Two of these are branches of the ophthalmic division of the Vth cranial nerve. They are the **lacrimal** and **frontal** nerves. The other nerve is the IVth cranial nerve, the **trochlear** nerve.

The ophthalmic division of the Vth nerve and its branches are purely sensory. The lacrimal branch of the Vth nerve carries sensory impulses from the conjunctiva and eyelids. The frontal branch of the Vth nerve divides into two branches (supraorbital and supratrochlear) and carries sensation from a wide area of skin extending from the side of the eye upwards over the scalp to the top of the head. The trochlear nerve, the IVth cranial nerve, is entirely motor. It is a small thread-like nerve and supplies only one muscle, the superior oblique.

Structures passing through the optic foramen and medial end of the superior orbital fissure must run within the cone of muscles. There are four nerves to consider. The **optic nerve** (the IInd cranial nerve) the **nasociliary** branch of the ophthalmic division of the

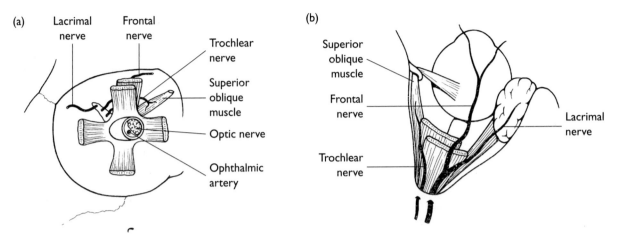

Figure 2.17 The lacrimal, frontal and trochlear nerves enter the orbital cavity through the superior orbital fissure outside the tendinous ring and above the levator palpebrae superioris.

Vth cranial nerve, the **oculomotor nerve** (III) and the **abducent** nerve (VI).

The optic nerve passes through the optic foramen and tendinous ring (Fig. 2.17(a)) to reach the eyeball about 3 mm medial to its posterior pole. This latter fact is important when examining the interior of the eye with an ophthalmoscope. The area of entrance of the optic nerve can be seen as a saucer-like depression called the **optic disc**.

The nasociliary branch is another branch of the ophthalmic division of the Vth cranial nerve and it enters the orbit within the cone of muscles (Fig. 2.18). Like the other two branches, the lacrimal and frontal,

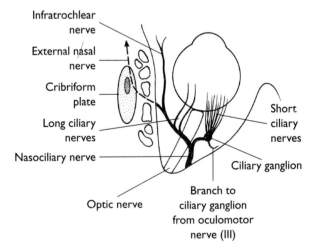

Figure 2.18 The nasociliary branch of the ophthalmic division of the trigeminal nerve (Vi) is a sensory nerve. It leaves the orbital cavity within the tendinous ring. Long and short ciliary nerves convey sensation from the eye, cornea and conjunctiva. Other branches innervate the bridge of the nose and forehead.

it is entirely sensory. It crosses *above* the optic nerve and passes towards the medial wall of the orbit, and here divides into branches that carry sensation from the surface and bridge of the nose, and from the air sinuses in the ethmoid bone. While in the orbit several important branches leave the main trunk of the naso-ciliary nerve. The **long ciliary nerves** are sensory nerves from the eyeball, but also carry sympathetic fibres to the eye (Fig. 2.20). Sympathetic activity causes the pupil to dilate. Some sensory neurons of the nasociliary nerve and some sympathetic neurons take another course to the eye through the **short ciliary nerves**. They pass first through a swelling known as the parasympathetic **ciliary ganglion**. Both the sympathetic fibres and the sensory fibres of course do this without synapsing. The sensory fibres simply continue through the ganglion to join up with the nasociliary nerve. The ciliary ganglion therefore appears to be suspended from the nasociliary nerve and hangs down just to the lateral side of the optic nerve (Fig. 2.18).

Like the nasociliary nerve, the oculomotor nerve also enters the orbit through the superior orbital fissure and within the cone of muscles attached to the tendinous ring (Fig. 2.19). The nerve divides into two divisions which supply all the extraocular muscles *except* superior oblique (which is supplied by the IVth cranial nerve) and the lateral rectus (which is supplied by the VIth cranial nerve). The oculomotor nerve also carries parasympathetic motor fibres from the brain. These fibres leave the nerve and jump into the ciliary ganglion. Here they synapse and postganglionic para-sympathetic fibres pass to the eye within the short

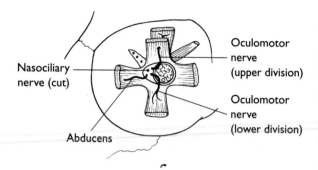

Figure 2.19   Both the abducens and the oculomotor nerves enter the orbital cavity within the tendinous ring. The abducens runs to the lateral rectus. The oculomotor nerve splits into upper and lower divisions which supply all the extraocular muscles except the superior oblique and the lateral rectus.

ciliary nerves. Figure 2.20 also gives a summary of the parasympathetic pathway through the ciliary ganglion and its connections. Activity of the parasympathetic fibres to the eye causes the pupil to constrict and the ciliary muscle to contract.

The abducent nerve (VI) is motor to only one muscle, the lateral rectus (Fig. 2.19). It passes through the medial end of the superior orbital fissure within the fibrous ring and quickly enters the lateral rectus muscle.

Clinically, it is important to test the movements of each eye as shown in Figure 2.16. In this way strabismus due to lesions of III, IV and VI may be detected. Some lesions, however, may also affect the *sympathetic* supply to the eye. Stimulation of sympathetic neurons to the eye causes the pupil to dilate.

Preganglionic neurons leave the thoracic spinal cord and ascend in the trunks to the upper cervical sympathetic ganglion, where they synapse. Postganglionic neurons climb along the carotid arteries and the ophthalmic branch to reach the orbit. Here they pass without synapse through the ciliary ganglion to the eye, or simply 'hitch-hike' along the long and short ciliary branches of the nasociliary nerve.

Since sympathetic fibres have such a long course it will readily be apparent that a lesion as far away as the apex of the lung in the thorax could affect the sympathetic trunk and the sympathetic supply to the eye. The pupil of the eye will then be unable to dilate and will remain small and constricted. Similarly, the parasympathetic neurons in the oculomotor nerve may also be compressed or injured. This is common during or following severe injury to the head. As a result of swelling and oedema of the brain, the pressure within the cranial cavity rises and the oculomotor nerve is easily compressed. The pupil on the side where there is raised pressure is therefore unable to constrict. It remains dilated and is sluggish or even unresponsive to a light shone into the eye.

Blood supply to the orbit

Arterial supply to the eye and orbit is via the **ophthalmic artery**. It enters the orbit below the optic

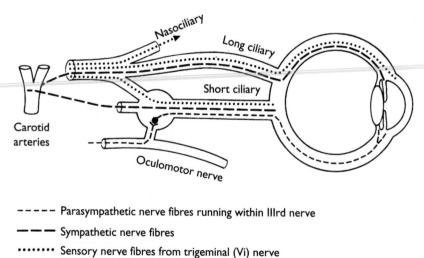

- - - - - Parasympathetic nerve fibres running within IIIrd nerve

— — — Sympathetic nerve fibres

• • • • • • • Sensory nerve fibres from trigeminal (Vi) nerve

Figure 2.20   Summary diagram of the sensory supply to the eye and of the parasympathetic and sympathetic nerve supply to the ciliary muscles and to the sphincter pupillae and dilator pupillae muscles.

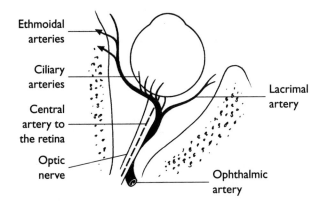

Figure 2.21 The most important branch of the ophthalmic artery is the central artery to the retina which is an end artery. For part of its course it runs within the substance of the optic nerve.

nerve through the optic foramen (Fig. 2.21). It then spirals around the lateral side of the optic nerve and supplies many branches to the muscles, eyelids, conjunctiva and other orbital structures. Branches of the ophthalmic artery supply the mucous membrane of the ethmoidal air sinuses and the root of the nose. The **anterior** and **posterior ethmoidal arteries** accompany branches of the nasociliary nerve through foramina, with the same names, out through the medial wall of the orbital cavity. Of course, the most important branch of the ophthalmic artery, the **central artery of the retina**, passes into the substance of the nerve itself and is carried into the eye with it. It is the only artery to the retina and blockage causes complete blindness.

Many veins drain the orbital cavity, mostly into the cavernous sinus. Many veins from the forehead and face drain back into the orbital cavity and so also drain to the cavernous sinus. But there are no valves in these veins and the direction of blood flow can reverse.

Applied anatomy of the eye and orbit

Fractured orbits are common and may involve the zygomatic bone. In this situation the patient complains of seeing double (diplopia). This is either because the suspensory ligament which supports the eye in the horizontal plane is no longer fixed in position or because the fractured bone now directly obstructs movements of the rectus muscles. The medial and inferior walls of the orbit are very thin and any blow to the eye that compresses the contents of the orbital cavity (for example, a hard ball striking the eyeball and orbital margin) is in danger of producing a 'blow-out' fracture of the orbital cavity.

Clinical conditions affecting the eyelids and eye are commonly encountered. Foreign bodies 'in the eye' are particularly common and often lodge under the upper eyelid in the superior fornix. Sometimes they injure the cornea and can cause corneal abrasion. Infections of the conjunctiva are called conjunctivitis. Sometimes an infection will ulcerate the cornea. Deeper infections are more serious when the iris and ciliary body are involved. These are called iridocyclitis. An opacity developing in the lens is called a cataract; when the lens becomes completely opaque it may need to be removed surgically to restore vision.

Squint or strabismus is the deviation of the eyes such that their axes are no longer parallel with each other. This of course excludes the normal convergence that occurs when the eyes adapt to very close work. A squint may be due to a lesion of one of the cranial nerves that supply the extraocular muscles, or it may be due to a localized problem with one of the muscles. A squint may be in any direction but commonly it is horizontal. When the eyes tend to look towards each other the squint is said to be convergent and when they look away from each other it is divergent.

It is important to understand what happens when there is a lesion of one of the cranial nerves supplying the extraocular muscles and eye. The oculomotor nerve (III) supplies the voluntary part of levator palpebrae superioris and all the other extraocular muscles except superior oblique and lateral rectus. It also carries parasympathetic fibres which constrict the pupil and act on the ciliary muscle during the accommodation reflex. It follows that in an ocular motor nerve lesion there is unopposed sympathetic action on the dilator pupillae muscle and the pupil remains dilated. Accommodation to close vision is also impossible. The upper eyelid closes because the involuntary portion of levator palpebrae superioris is unable to raise the lid on its own. There is unopposed action of the lateral rectus muscle which abducts the eye. In this position the superior oblique muscle is aligned across the equator of the eye and can only rotate or 'intort' the globe. Many oculomotor nerve lesions are only partial and may be more difficult to spot than a complete IIIrd nerve lesion.

A lesion of the VIth nerve (abducens) presents with the patient unable to abduct the eye to the side of the lesion. Attempts to do this lead to double vision as the unaffected eye adducts but the affected eye remains centrally placed. IVth nerve (trochlear) lesions are extremely rare on their own. They are usually picked up because the patient complains they are unable to look down towards the nose, which leads to difficulty walking down stairs. With the eye medially placed the superior oblique muscle is aligned along its visual axis and so, being inserted behind the equator of the globe, is perfectly positioned to depress the eyeball. This is not possible in a IVth nerve lesion.

Horner's syndrome results when there is disruption of the sympathetic trunk. This may result, for example, from a lung tumour invading the trunk either in the thorax or at the neck of the first rib, or it may even result from a poorly placed local anaesthetic in the neck or mouth. There is unopposed parasympathetic activity which results in a constricted pupil and a hot flushed dry face and neck since it is sympathetic fibres which innervate sweat glands and are vasoconstrictor in action. Drooping of the upper eyelid also occurs because of the loss of sympathetic innervation to levator palpebrae superioris. The voluntary fibres to this muscle from the ocular motor nerve (III) are insufficient on their own to raise the lid completely.

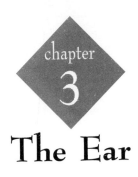

chapter

3

The Ear

The external ear

The external ear consists of the **auricle**, or **pinna**, and the **external acoustic** or **auditory meatus** (Fig. 3.1). Much of the auricle has a supporting elastic fibrocartilaginous framework with skin firmly attached to this. Its surface is thrown into numerous complex depressions and folds which collect sound waves and allow us to discriminate their direction more easily. The outermost rim of the auricle is called the **helix** and this runs into the **lobule** below. The lobule is fleshy and has no fibrocartilaginous support. The inner rim of the auricle is called the **antihelix** and this encircles a deeper concave portion of the auricle called the **concha** (since it looks like the interior of a shell). Hearing aid moulds are carefully constructed to fit into the concha and external meatus with an air-tight seal here. Anteriorly, at the entrance to the external auditory meatus, the **tragus** projects laterally a little, as a spur of elastic fibrocartilage.

Both the external acoustic meatus and the membrane of its inner end, the **tympanic membrane**, may be examined with the aid of an auriscope. In the newborn child the external auditory meatus is very short, and great care is exercised when conducting such an examination. In adults the outer third of the meatus is cartilaginous, and only the inner section is walled by bone. Most of the bone is formed by the **tympanic plate** of the temporal bone. The external auditory meatus forms an S-shaped curve, first curving anteriorly and then posteriorly, finally veering anteroinferiorly to reach the tympanic membrane. This membrane is not set at right angles to the meatus but is placed obliquely so that the anterior wall and floor of the meatus are longer than the roof and posterior wall. To straighten the meatus for auroscopic examination the auricle must be pulled upwards and backwards.

The appearance of the normal tympanic membrane during auroscopic examination is characteristic (Fig. 3.2). Certain parts of the **malleus**, one of the middle ear ossicles, shine through the membrane. The **long handle** of this bone is attached to the inner surface of the membrane and can be seen as a streak passing downwards and backwards to a point just below its centre. At the upper end of the handle a small **lateral process** of the bone creates a prominence on the membrane. Anterior and posterior folds extend upwards from the upper end of the handle to the periphery of the membrane. Enclosed between these folds is a **flaccid part** of the membrane, which is particularly vascular. The tympanic membrane is

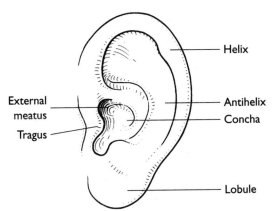

Figure 3.1 The most important named parts of the pinna, or auricle, of the external ear.

Helix

External meatus

Tragus

Antihelix

Concha

Lobule

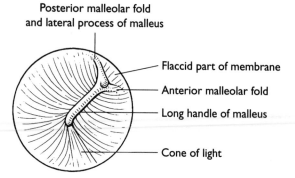

Posterior malleolar fold
and lateral process of malleus

— Flaccid part of membrane

— Anterior malleolar fold

— Long handle of malleus

— Cone of light

Figure 3.2 On auroscopic examination, the long handle of the malleus shines through the tympanic membrane. Two malleolar folds enclose a vascular area of the membrane above and a cone of light is reflected across the inferior portion of the membrane.

drawn inwards towards the handle of the malleus so that the outer surface of the membrane is concave. Light reflected from the auroscope produces a cone of reflected light in the anteroinferior quadrant of the membrane.

The external auditory meatus and the external aspect of the tympanic membrane receive sensory nerve fibres from both the vagus nerve (the Xth cranial nerve) and the trigeminal nerve (the Vth cranial nerve).

The middle ear

The middle ear or **tympanic cavity** is a small air-filled space within the petrous temporal bone (Fig. 3.3). It communicates with the pharynx in front through the **auditory tube** (sometimes called the **Eustachian tube**

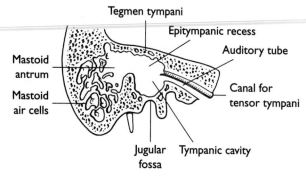

Tegmen tympani

Epitympanic recess

Auditory tube

Mastoid antrum

Mastoid air cells

Canal for tensor tympani

Jugular fossa   Tympanic cavity

Figure 3.3 An oblique section through the tympanic cavity of the middle ear, mastoid antrum and mastoid process of the temporal bone. (After Hollinshead WH (1982) *Anatomy for Surgeons*. Philadelphia: Harper and Row.)

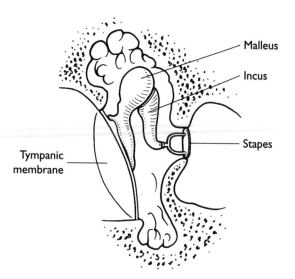

Malleus

Incus

Stapes

Tympanic membrane

Figure 3.4 The malleus, incus and stapes are joined to each other by synovial joints. Pressure per unit area is 20 times greater at the footplate of the stapes than at the tympanic membrane.

or **pharyngotympanic tube**) and with the **mastoid antrum** behind. The upper part of the cavity is expanded into an **epitympanic recess**. The middle ear contains a chain of three ossicles (small bones) connecting the tympanic membrane to a membrane of the inner ear (Fig. 3.4). These transmit vibrations across the cavity from the external to the internal ear. There is then a mechanical coupling between the vibrations of the tympanic membrane and the vibrations of fluid within the inner ear.

Although the tympanic cavity is irregular in shape, it is more easily understood if it is described as having lateral, medial, anterior and posterior walls, a roof and a floor. You will get the general idea of this if you look for a moment at Figure 3.5. Overall, the cavity is about the size of a hearing aid battery and has similar proportions. The lateral wall is formed by the tympanic membrane. The medial wall is the bone of the inner ear, and it presents several eminences and grooves produced by structures within the bone of the inner ear. The **promontory** is a rounded elevation on the medial wall produced by the underlying **cochlea**. Just behind this are two openings in the bone which lead into the bony cavities of the inner ear. The upper opening is the **fenestra vestibuli** or **oval window**. It is closed in life by a part of one of the middle ear ossicles, the **stapes**. The lower opening is the **fenestra cochleae** or **round window**, and it is closed over by a secondary tympanic membrane.

The anterior wall of the tympanic cavity leads to

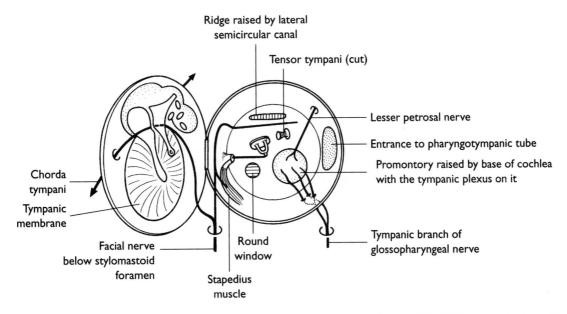

Ridge raised by lateral
semicircular canal

Tensor tympani (cut)

Lesser petrosal nerve

Entrance to pharyngotympanic tube

Promontory raised by base of cochlea
with the tympanic plexus on it

Chorda
tympani

Tympanic
membrane

Facial nerve
below stylomastoid
foramen

Round
window

Stapedius
muscle

Tympanic branch of
glossopharyngeal nerve

Figure 3.5 Diagrammatic representation of the middle ear cavity. (After: Green JH and Silver PHS (1981) *An Introduction to Human Anatomy.* New York: Oxford Medical Publications.)

two canals, the auditory tube and a canal for the **tensor tympani muscle** (Figs 3.3 and 3.5). The auditory tube is the lower and larger of the two, and passes obliquely towards the pharynx. The canal is at first within the petrous part of the temporal bone, but is continued to the pharynx as a cartilaginous tube. The tube acts as a protective mechanism for the middle ear by allowing pressure to be equalized on the two sides of the tympanic membrane at all times. The tube is opened during swallowing and yawning, and the cartilaginous part is related to several muscles which are active then. The mucous membrane of the auditory tube is supplied by the glossopharyngeal nerve (IXth cranial nerve). Above the auditory tube is a canal for the tensor tympani muscle. This small muscle enters the tympanic cavity and gives rise to a delicate tendon which changes direction to reach its insertion into the handle of the malleus. It does this by passing around a small bony pulley called the **processus trochleariformis**. The canal conducting the internal carotid artery through the skull base is related to the anterior wall of the middle ear, with only a thin lamina of bone separating the two.

In the posterior wall of the tympanic cavity an opening, or **aditus**, leads from the epitympanic recess into the mastoid antrum. A small pyramidal eminence containing the **stapedius muscle** is found on the posterior wall below the aditus. The tendon of this muscle emerges through the summit of the pyramid, and travels from here to its insertion into the stapes. The roof of the tympanic cavity is thin and formed by part of the petrous temporal bone called the **tegmen tympani**. Above this is the temporal lobe of the brain. The floor of the tympanic cavity is related to the jugular foramen and the internal jugular vein.

The three ossicles, the malleus, incus and stapes, contained within the tympanic cavity are united by synovial joints (Fig. 3.4). The malleus is said to look like a hammer, its head lying in the epitympanic recess. It is held in place there by ligaments. The handle of the malleus is firmly attached to the inner surface of the tympanic membrane. The head of the incus articulates with the malleus at a saddle-shaped synovial joint. The incus has a short process that is anchored to the wall of the epitympanic recess and a long process that articulates with the head of the stapes at a tiny synovial ball and socket joint. The long process of the incus runs downwards and backwards in the middle ear cavity in parallel with the long handle of the malleus. The footplate of the stapes fits into and closes the fenestra vestibuli, or oval window, of the inner ear. The stapedius muscle attaches to the neck of the stapes.

The mastoid antrum and mastoid process

The mastoid antrum is an air sinus within the petrous part of the temporal bone and it lies behind the middle ear. It is the only paranasal air sinus to be well developed at birth, although the mastoid process of the temporal bone is *not* formed at this time. The mastoid antrum is important clinically because of the possibility of spread of infection into it from the middle ear. The aditus in the anterior wall of the mastoid antrum leads into the epitympanic recess. Posteriorly, the mastoid antrum is related to the sigmoid sinus, and here the bone may be quite thin. The roof of the antrum is related to the brain. The medial wall of the antrum is related to the posterior semicircular canal.

The mastoid process itself does not begin to develop until the second year of life. At this time air cells gradually extend into it. The cavities are continuous with the air-containing mastoid antrum and the tympanic cavity. Occasionally, air cells are found in other parts of the petrous temporal bone. A group of air cells often extends as far as the apex of the petrous temporal bone. The mucous membrane of the mastoid air cells is supplied partly by the mandibular division of the trigeminal nerve (Vth cranial nerve) via the **nervus spinosus** which passes up to them via the foramen spinosum. Glossopharyngeal nerve (IX) fibres from the middle ear cavity also contribute.

The inner ear

The deeper part of the petrous temporal bone contains a series of cavities and canals called the **bony labyrinth** (Fig. 3.6). The bony cavities are filled with a fluid called **perilymph**. The organs of hearing and balance fit inside this complex network as the **membranous labyrinth** (Fig. 3.7), and these in turn contain **endolymph**. The membranous labyrinth is tied down or anchored to the bony labyrinth at several points and so is not afloat within it.

The bony labyrinth

The bony labyrinth consists of a centrally placed cavity called the **vestibule** which communicates

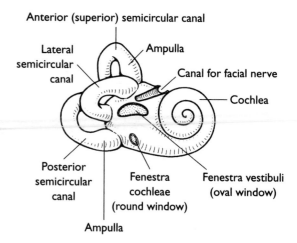

Figure 3.6   The bony labyrinth consists of the vestibule from which the three semicircular canals emerge poseriorly and the cochlea, which is positioned anterior to the vestibule. The fenestra vestibuli (oval window) is closed by the footplate of the stapes and the fenestra cochleae (round window) by a secondary tympanic membrane.

behind with three bony **semicircular canals**. In front, the vestibule leads to a curled bony canal, the **cochlea**. The bony labyrinth contains perilymph whose composition closely resembles that of cerebrospinal fluid. A passageway or **aqueduct of the cochlea** passes through the petrous temporal bone from the cochlea to the jugular foramen and into the subarachnoid space. It is said that there is a flow of cerebrospinal fluid along this duct. It is likely, however, that perilymph also originates as a

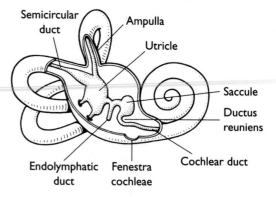

Figure 3.7   The membranous labyrinth lies within the bony labyrinth and is surrounded by perilymph. Semicircular ducts pass from the utricle into the bony semicircular canals. The cochlear duct passes from the saccule via the ductus reuniens into the cochlea. Endolymph produced within the membranous labyrinth also enters the endolymphatic duct and is eventually resorbed into the venous system through dura at a point on the posterior aspect of the petrous temporal bone.

transudate from blood vessels in the walls of the bony labyrinth. Perilymph may be removed through the aqueduct of the cochlea, but other mechanisms of removal are also likely. The fenestra vestibuli is an opening on the lateral wall of the vestibule, and is closed in life by the footplate of the stapes. Movement of the stapes therefore transmits pressure waves to the perilymph of the vestibule.

The cochlea

The cochlea is a sinuous tunnel which runs forwards from the cavity of the vestibule (Fig. 3.7). It resembles the shell of a snail, with approximately two and three-quarters turns. The apex of the cochlea, the **cupula**, lies deep to the medial wall of the tympanic cavity. The first turn of the cochlea raises a bulge called the **promontory** on the medial wall of the middle ear cavity. The cochlea is wound around a central axis called the **modiolus** (Fig. 3.8). Its canal is partially divided by a **bony spiral lamina**, which projects from the central column into the canal. The division of the canal of the cochlea is completed by a **basilar membrane** which stretches from the edge of the spiral lamina to the outer wall of the canal. The canal of the cochlea is thus completely divided into a **scala** (staircase) **vestibuli** above and a **scala tympani** below. The two canals are continuous through a gap at the apex of the cochlea called the **helicotrema**. Vibrations in the

perilymph, created by movement of the footplate of the stapes, travel along the scala vestibuli to the apex of the cochlea. From here vibrations pass through the helicotrema into the scala tympani, and then downwards to the base of the cochlea and the fenestra cochleae. This is closed over by the secondary tympanic membrane. Thus, movements occur at this membrane which are opposite in direction to those of the footplate of the stapes. In this way, pressure in the inner ear perilymph does not become excessive.

The semicircular canals

Semicircular canals lead posteriorly from the vestibule and are named **anterior** (or superior), **posterior** and **lateral** (Figs 3.6 and 3.9). At one end, each of them has a dilation or **ampulla** which contains organs sensitive to body movement. The anterior and posterior canals are vertically placed. The posterior canal lies in the long axis of the petrous temporal bone and the anterior canal lies at right angles to this axis. The anterior canal lies at a higher level than the posterior canal when the head is held in the horizontal position, and this is why it is often called the 'superior' canal. In fact the anterior or superior semicircular canal raises a bony eminence on the anterior aspect of the petrous temporal bone in the middle cranial fossa called the

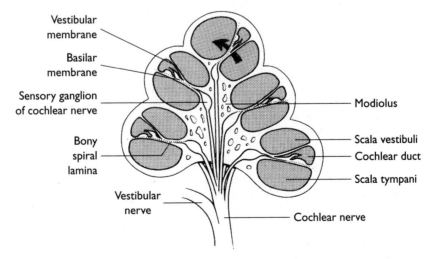

Figure 3.8 The cochlear duct is enclosed by the basilar and vestibular membranes which both lie between the scala vestibuli and the scala tympani in the coils of the cochlea. At the helicotrema (arrowed) the scala vestibuli and the scala tympani are continuous with each other. The central modiolus of the cochlea contains the cell bodies of the sensory nerve fibres of the cochlear part of the VIIIth cranial nerve.

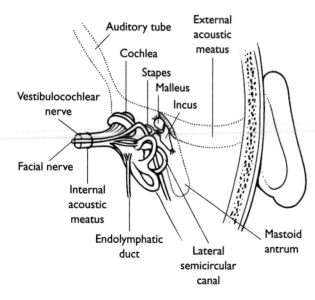

Figure 3.9 The basal turn of the cochlea raises a promontory on the medial wall of the middle ear cavity. The posterior semicircular canal lies in the axis of the petrous temporal bone and the anterior (or superior) semicircular canal lies at right angles to it. The lateral semicircular canal lies in the horizontal plane.

arcuate eminence. The lateral semicircular canal lies horizontally.

The membranous labyrinth

The cavities and canals of the bony labyrinth contain a series of membranous sacs and tubes filled with endolymph (Fig. 3.7). This membranous labyrinth is smaller than the cavities and canals of the bony labyrinth. Two sacs of endolymph lie within the vestibule, the **utricle** behind and the **saccule** in front. **Semicircular ducts** are continuous posteriorly with the utricle and lie within the bony semicircular canals. In front, the saccule communicates with the **cochlear duct**, which lies within the bony cochlear canal. A blind-ending sac, the **endolymphatic duct**, arises from both the utricle and saccule. This duct extends through the petrous bone in the bony **aqueduct of the vestibule** and comes to lie against the dura in the posterior cranial fossa on the posterior aspect of the petrous temporal bone. The dura in this position covers over a hole in the bone here. At this point endolymph is resorbed back into the circulating blood stream from the endolymphatic duct via a vascular plexus in the specialized epithelial cells here.

The saccule, utricle and semicircular canals

The saccule is joined to the duct of the cochlea in front by the **ductus reuniens**. Both utricle and saccule also contain specialized neuroepithelium sensitive to the pull of gravity. Part of the wall of the utricle is thickened by this specialized organ, called the **macula**. A similar thickening is found in the wall of the saccule, the macula of the saccule. This is set at right angles to the macula of the utricle. Three semicircular ducts occupy the semicircular canals of the bony labyrinth, and open into the utricle. Near the orifices, the ducts are dilated as **ampullae**, and each contains a projection called an **ampullary crest**.

The maculae of the utricle and saccule signal *alterations in the position* of the head with reference to the pull of gravity. Much of the information from these organs produces appropriate alterations in muscle tone throughout the body. The supporting muscles, muscles of the neck and muscles concerned with eye movement are particularly affected. The maculae are therefore referred to as the organs of static balance.

The epithelium of the maculae and of the ampullary crests is composed of hair cells and supporting cells. The bases of most hair cells are associated with nerve terminals belonging to the afferent fibres of the vestibular nerve. A gelatinous mass or **otolithic membrane** overlies each macula and it contains crystalline bodies or **otoconia**. Alterations in the position of the head, relative to the line of gravity, are reflected in the drag of the otolithic membrane on the sensitive hair cells.

The ampullary crests of the semicircular canals signal *angular acceleration* of the head rather than static balance. The ampullary crests also are covered with a gelatinous dome-shaped **cupula**. This rests on the surface of each ampullary crest (Fig. 3.10). The minute **stereocilia** of sensitive hair cells on the ampullary crest are embedded into the substance of the cupula. The cupula, in fact, entirely blocks off the flow of endolymph around the semicircular canals, but drag and currents in the endolymph, set up during movement, press against it and draw the cupula from side to side. This stimulates the hair cells, which discharge nerve impulses accordingly. Vestibular nerve fibres have a continuous basal discharge. Bending the cupula to one side increases the frequency of discharge and to the opposite side decreases the frequency.

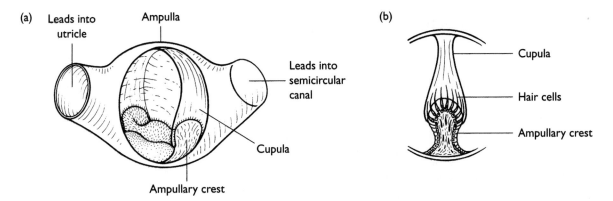

Figure 3.10 Within each ampulla (a) of the semicircular canals there is an ampullary crest from which sensitive stereocilia of the hair cells of the crest protrude. These are embedded into a gelatinous cupula (b). The cupula completely occludes the lumen of the semicircular canal but fluid pressure against it, following angular movements of the head, distorts the stereocilia and triggers nerve impulses that pass to the vestibular part of the VIIIth cranial nerve.

The cochlear duct

The **cochlear duct** is a spirally arranged tube concerned with hearing. It starts below at the ductus reuniens and spirals to a closed end near the apex of the cochlea. The floor of the duct is the basilar membrane which stretches from the spiral bony lamina to the outer wall of the cochlear canal (Fig. 3.11). The roof is formed by vestibular membrane, which also extends from the lamina to the outer surface of the cochlear canal. The cochlear duct is therefore triangular in cross-section. Above the attachment of the basilar membrane, the outer wall of the cochlear duct presents a spiral prominence. The epithelium above the prominence is highly vascular and called the **stria vascularis.** This is thought to be concerned with the production of endolymph as well as with the maintenance of its ionic composition.

The specialized receptor organ for hearing lies within the cochlear duct on the basilar membrane, and is called the **spiral organ of Corti.** It is composed of several parts. Inner and outer hair cells sit on the basilar membrane. These cells form pillars that slope towards each other and create a triangular **tunnel of Corti** between them. The outer 'hairs', or stereocilia, of the hair cells are embedded in a fibrogelatinous membrane which extends above them all and is called the **tectorial membrane.** The stereocilia of the inner hair cells are free of the tectorial membrane.

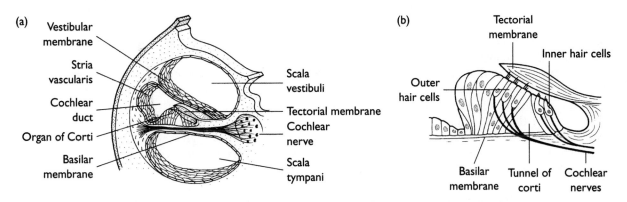

Figure 3.11 Stereocilia of the outer hair cells of the organ of Corti are embedded into the fibrogelatinous membrana tectoria above them. Shear between the basilar membrane and the tectorial membrane, set up by pressure waves in the scala vestibuli and scala tympani, triggers nerve impulses from the hair cells which pass into the cochlear nerve fibres.

Summary of the mechanisms of hearing

It is now possible to summarize the basic mechanism of the sense of hearing. Sound vibrations are collected by the pinna and transmitted through the external acoustic meatus to the tympanic membrane. From here movements of the ossicles transmit the vibrations towards the inner ear. In this way the force per unit area at the footplate of the stapes is amplified some 20 times. The stapedius and tensor tympani muscles help by dampening excess vibrations. They do this by stiffening the chain of ossicles. Vibration of the stapes creates pressure waves in the fluid within the vestibule. These waves are conducted via the perilymph of the scala vestibuli and the scala tympani to the basilar and vestibular membranes that lie between them. Naturally, the cochlear system cannot be closed off completely, or the pressure within it would rise to excess. Therefore every inward excursion of the oval window produces a pressure wave through the scala vestibuli, around the apex of the cochlea, through the scala tympani and is then dissipated as an outward movement of the secondary tympanic membrane of the round window.

The basilar membrane actually increases in width from its base to its apex and also increases in stiffness. Low sound frequencies set up vibrations in the whole of the basilar membrane. With increasing sound frequencies, however, the maximum amplitude of so-called 'travelling waves' set up along the basilar membrane moves progressively from the apex to the basal end of the cochlear duct. The amount and extent of vibration in the cochlear duct depends on the pitch and volume of the sound waves. The duct contains the special sense organs that respond to these pressure waves. The simplistic explanation for the way we perceive sounds of different pitch and loudness is that shear in the stereocilia of the hair cells occurs with increasing or decreasing magnitude at different positions between the basal and vestibular lamina along the length of the cochlear duct. Impulses from the hair cells are carried towards the spiral ganglion cell bodies which lie in the modiolus. From here neurons pass onwards as the cochlear part of the VIIIth nerve.

The vestibulocochlear nerve

The VIIIth cranial nerve, the **vestibulocochlear nerve**, carries impulses both from the organs of hearing and from the organs of balance to the brain. Hair cells in the cochlear duct, deformed by vibrations, set up impulses which are conducted through cochlear fibres of the vestibulocochlear nerve. The sensory cell bodies of these fibres are found in the spiral ganglion. Vestibular fibres carry impulses set up by movements of the sensitive hair cells both in the maculae and in the ampullary crests.

The facial nerve in the petrous temporal bone

At this point it is important to understand that another cranial nerve, the VIIth or **facial nerve**, also uses the internal acoustic meatus to enter the petrous temporal bone. It then bypasses the ear cavities within its own tunnel. So, for a short distance, the VIIth and VIIIth nerves travel together. The VIIth nerve is on its way to supply the muscles of the face and we will discuss it further when we study this region. For now, we will simply outline its course through the petrous temporal bone.

The facial nerve passes laterally along the internal acoustic meatus until it reaches the medial wall of the middle ear cavity (Fig. 3.12). The sensory fibres within the facial nerve have their cells bodies here in a ganglion called the **geniculate ganglion**. The nerve then turns a right angle backwards and runs along the top of the medial wall of the middle ear cavity in its own bony canal. On reaching the back of the medial wall it turns another right angle downwards in its canal and eventually runs out of the petrous temporal bone and skull through the **stylomastoid foramen**.

While in its tunnel in the petrous temporal bone the facial nerve gives off several branches. Two **petrosal nerves** run forwards through the petrous temporal bone and we will describe their functions later. Two branches of the facial nerve need more careful attention at this point because they relate directly to structures we have already discussed. The first of these is a branch that enters the cavity of the middle ear and supplies the tiny stapedius

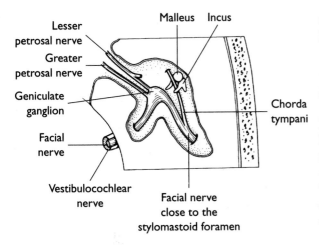

Lesser petrosal nerve

Greater petrosal nerve

Geniculate ganglion

Facial nerve

Vestibulocochlear nerve

Malleus   Incus

Chorda tympani

Facial nerve close to the stylomastoid foramen

Figure 3.12   The facial nerve enters the internal acoustic meatus in company with the vestibulocochlear nerve and the labyrinthine artery. At the geniculate ganglion, the facial nerve gives off the greater petrosal nerve (which runs anteriorly through bone with the lesser petrosal nerve). The facial nerve continues posteriorly and then runs down to the stylomastoid foramen. Within the middle ear cavity the facial nerve gives off the motor nerve to stapedius and the chorda tympani.

muscle. It is therefore called the **nerve to stapedius**. You will recall that there are two small muscles in the middle ear attached to bony ossicles, the stapedius and tensor tympani. The action of both muscles is to stabilize the excursions of the ossicles. They prevent you dislocating your ear ossicles when you go to discos. But while the stapedius is supplied by its branch of the VIIth cranial nerve, the tensor tympani is supplied by the Vth cranial nerve. Paralysis of the stapedius muscle leads to **hyperacusia**, an excessive acuteness of hearing.

The second branch of the facial nerve that needs attention now is the **chorda tympani**. This branch is given off in the bony facial canal as the facial nerve approaches the stylomastoid foramen. The chorda tympani then runs forwards, high up over the tympanic membrane and handle of the malleus, and eventually leaves the skull (Fig. 3.5). The chorda tympani carries taste fibres from the tongue and secretor motor fibres to the salivary glands in

the floor of the mouth, and we will return to it again later on.

Applied anatomy of the ear

Minor infections, lodged foreign bodies and accumulations of 'wax' in the external auditory meatus are frequent causes of complaint and can each cause pain and lead to more serious complications. Infections in the middle ear cavity occur frequently, especially in children, and can spread to the mastoid air cells. They often originate in the pharynx and track up the auditory tube to the middle ear. Children with cleft palate are therefore especially susceptible to middle ear infections. Persistent infections can lead to deafness. The tympanic membrane appears red and swollen, and the cone of light is not visible in middle ear infections. Occasionally, it becomes necessary to incise the tympanic membrane to drain the middle ear cavity. The superior half of the tympanic membrane is very vascular and the chorda tympani runs over the membrane here. The handle of the malleus is attached to the upper half of the membrane also. The least vascular portion of the tympanic membrane, and one that avoids all these important structures, is the posteroinferior quadrant. It is here that incisions in the tympanic membrane are made.

There are many causes of vertigo and deafness. Labyrinthitis or inflammation of the membranous labyrinth is one cause of vertigo. Excess production of endolymph that leads to increased pressure and subsequent degeneration of hair cells in the maculae is another (Menière's disease). Syringing wax out of the external auditory meatus with water that is much below or above body temperature will also induce a movement of endolymph that results in dizziness. Deafness may result either from damage to the vestibulocochlear nerve (VIII) or from mechanical disruption to sound transmission through the chain of ossicles somewhere between the tympanic membrane and the oval window. Congenital fixation of the stapes to the oval window is a case in point here.

Summary and Revision of the Intracranial Region, Orbit, Eye and Ear

First read through the summaries of the cranial nerves we have just studied in this first section. Be sure you understand their course, their actions and how you would test their functions. Use Figure 4.1 to help you as you read through the summaries. Some of the multiple choice questions that follow require a knowledge of facts given in these summaries. To bring together what you have learned about the intracranial region, the eye and the ear, go through the multiple choice questions at the end of this chapter. For each **stem,** any one of the five answers (A)–(E) may be either correct or incorrect. You may choose to do them all on one occasion or you may choose to do only alternate questions at your first attempt. Many of these questions are quite searching. A score of around 50% correct would be very reasonable at your first attempt. We expect you to have to refer back to the text to improve your score on subsequent attempts. In so doing you will improve your understanding of head and neck anatomy.

Summary of cranial nerves I, II, III, IV, Vi, VI, VII and VIII

Cranial nerve I

The olfactory nerve and bulb may be considered an extension of the brain. Some 20 olfactory nerve bundles pass to the olfactory bulb through the cribriform plate of the ethmoid in the anterior cranial fossa from the roof of the nose. Olfactory nerves only innervate the upper part of the nasal cavity. Loss of the sense of smell, anosmia, may be a clue to a fracture involving the cribriform plate or may be indicative of, for example, a

neuroma or meningioma compressing the olfactory bulb or tract. Anosmia is, however, common following a cold or upper respiratory tract infection. Asking patients to identify strong smells, such as coffee or chocolate, through each nostril in turn is a way of testing the olfactory nerve.

Cranial nerve II

The optic nerves are concerned with vision. They pass from the back of the eye through the orbit and then through the optic canal in the sphenoid bone. Nerve impulses from the lateral part of the retina run to the visual cortex of the same side. Nerve impulses from the nasal side of the retina cross to the other side in the optic chiasma. The optic chiasma lies in front of the pituitary stalk and between the terminal parts of both internal carotid arteries. Bitemporal hemianopia results when a pituitary tumour presses on the centre of the optic chiasma. The nasal parts of the retina which receive light from the temporal fields are insensitive to light. Nasal hemianopia results if there is pressure to the side of the optic chiasma. Visual field defects need to be described and plotted with care for each eye when testing the optic nerve.

Cranial nerve III

The oculomotor nerve supplies all the extrinsic muscles of the eye except lateral rectus, superior oblique and an involuntary part of levator palpebrae superioris. It passes from the front of the midbrain, between the posterior cerebral and superior cerebellar arteries and into the cleft of dura between the free edge of the tentorium and the dura over the petroclinoid ligament. It runs forwards in the lateral wall of the cavernous sinus and through the superior orbital fissure (within the tendinous ring) to enter the orbit. The muscles it supplies can be tested by asking a subject to look from side to side and then to look up and down with the eye placed alternately medially and laterally.

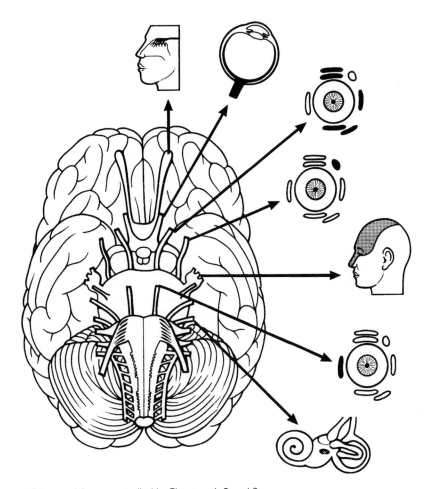

Figure 4.1 Summary of the cranial nerves studied in Chapters 1, 2 and 3.

Cranial nerve IV

The trochlear nerve is a small thread-like nerve that arises from the back of the midbrain. It then runs forwards under the free edge of the tentorium and passes beneath and lateral to the IIIrd nerve to enter the dura of the lateral wall of the cavernous sinus. The trochlear nerve enters the orbit through the outer part of the superior orbital fissure (outside the tendinous ring). It then passes medially to supply the superior oblique muscle. It can be tested by asking a subject to look towards the nose and then downwards.

Cranial nerve Vi

The trigeminal nerve leaves the anterolateral surface of the pons and passes forwards to the petrous crest over which it runs with an extension of dura and arachnoid from the posterior cranial fossa. Here in a depression on the apex of the petrous bone, in Meckel's cave, is the sensory trigeminal ganglion. Three large sensory divisions extend from the ganglion, and the motor part of the nerve now joins the mandibular or third division. The first division, the ophthalmic, runs through the lateral wall of the cavernous sinus. It divides into frontal, lacrimal and nasociliary

branches. These are sensory to the conjunctiva, the skin of the upper eyelid, the bridge of the nose and the forehead, as well as to the cornea and sclera through the long and short ciliary branches. The second division, or maxillary division, also runs in the lateral wall of the cavernous sinus. It is the sensory nerve to the mid-face, nasal cavity and palate as well as to the lower eyelid and associated conjunctiva via the infraorbital nerve. We will summarize its branches in more detail after we have studied the nose and mid-face. The sensory branches of these divisions of the nerve can be tested for touch, temperature, pressure and pain, where appropriate and by appropriate means, over the dermatomes on the skin of the forehead and face.

Cranial nerve VI

The abducent nerve leaves the brain from lower anterior aspect of the pons and therefore runs a long way up the clivus before it pierces the dura. It then runs under the petroclinoid ligament and into the cavernous sinus. Its long course makes it vulnerable to injury. It accompanies the internal carotid artery through the cavernous sinus and enters the orbit through the superior orbital fissure (within the fibrous ring). The abducent nerve supplies the lateral rectus muscle. The action of this muscle can be tested by asking a subject to follow and look at an object held out to the edge of the temporal field of view with the eye of the same side.

Cranial nerve VII

The facial nerve emerges between the pons and medulla and passes laterally into the internal acoustic meatus. It is eventually destined to supply the muscles of facial expression. The facial nerve continues laterally in the internal acoustic meatus until it approaches the medial wall of the middle ear cavity. Here its sensory root has a ganglion, called the geniculate ganglion, which contains cell bodies of these sensory nerve fibres. The facial nerve turns posteriorly at this point (the genu) in a bony canal and runs towards the posterior wall of the middle ear cavity. It then travels down the posterior wall, still in its own bony canal, and leaves the skull through the stylomastoid foramen. The facial nerve gives off the greater superficial petrosal nerve close to the geniculate ganglion. It gives a branch to the stapedius muscle in the middle ear cavity and gives off the chorda tympani just before it leaves the skull through the stylomastoid foramen. The chorda tympani runs forwards over the handle of the malleus and the tympanic membrane. It leaves the skull base through the petrotympanic fissure and then immediately joins the lingual nerve. We will describe the course of the facial nerve through the face and the chorda tympani into the floor of the mouth later.

Cranial nerve VIII

The vestibulocochlear nerve is the nerve of hearing and balance. It emerges close to the facial nerve between the pons and medulla and passes into the internal acoustic meatus. Here it runs with the facial nerve and labyrinthine artery (another end artery like the central artery to the retina) towards the cochlea and vestibular apparatus. The nerve fibres of the cochlear division have their sensory ganglia in the modiolus of the cochlea. The nerve fibres of the vestibular division have their sensory ganglia in the internal acoustic meatus. A simple test of vestibular function is to ask the subject to stand with feet together and to close their eyes. The subject will sway or fall to the side of any recent vestibular lesion. Tests for hearing impairment are very complex but simple tests with a tuning fork will distinguish between sensorineural deafness and deafness due to conduction between the external auditory meatus and the footplate of the stapes. Normally, air-conducted sound is louder than bone-conducted sound. If the sound-conducting pathway is damaged then bone conduction is better than air conduction. A tuning fork placed first on the mastoid process and then beside the ear will allow one to distinguish this.

Multiple Choice Questions on the Intracranial Region, Eye and Ear

1. In the skull at birth:
(A) the anterior fontanelle has already closed
(B) the mastoid antrum (or air sinus) is well developed
(C) the tympanic membrane is closer to the surface than in the adult skull
(D) there is a midline suture through the frontal bone
(E) the frontal and maxillary air sinuses are well developed

A___ B___ C___ D___ E___

2. The parietal bone:
(A) forms a suture with the occipital bone
(B) is grooved by meningeal vessels on its inner aspect
(C) forms a suture with the zygomatic bone
(D) contains erythropoietic tissue within its diploë
(E) is grooved by the transverse venous sinus on its inner aspect

A___ B___ C___ D___ E___

3. The falx cerebri:
(A) is attached to the crista galli
(B) contains the straight sinus at its attachment to the tentorium cerebelli
(C) is attached to the anterior clinoid process
(D) lies in the midline between the two cerebral hemispheres
(E) has the superior sagittal sinus in its upper margin

A___ B___ C___ D___ E___

4. The tentorium cerebelli:
(A) has a free edge which attaches to the posterior clinoid process
(B) contains the transverse venous sinus in its lateral margin
(C) attaches to the lesser wing of the sphenoid bone
(D) supports the weight of the cerebellum
(E) has a close relationship with the trochlear nerve

A___ B___ C___ D___ E___

5. The cavernous sinus:
(A) lies in the anterior cranial fossa
(B) receives veins from the orbit
(C) has the internal carotid artery passing through its substance
(D) has the abducent nerve (VI) in its lateral wall
(E) communicates with both the petrosal venous sinuses

A___ B___ C___ D___ E___

6. The middle cranial fossa:
(A) has the foramen rotundum leading out of it anteriorly
(B) supports the frontal lobes of the brain
(C) has the jugular foramen in its floor
(D) has the internal acoustic meatus in its lateral wall
(E) is formed partly by the temporal bone

A___ B___ C___ D___ E___

7. The posterior cranial fossa:
(A) contains the sigmoid venous sinuses
(B) contains the stylomastoid foramen
(C) contains the inferior petrosal sinuses
(D) contains the terminal parts of both vertebral arteries
(E) contains the foramen spinosum

A___ B___ C___ D___ E___

8. The foramen ovale:
(A) passes through the greater wing of the sphenoid bone
(B) transmits the mandibular division of the trigeminal nerve (Vi)
(C) transmits the maxillary division of the trigeminal nerve (Vii)
(D) transmits the lesser superficial petrosal nerve
(E) transmits the facial nerve (VII)

A___ B___ C___ D___ E___

9. Concerning the middle meningeal artery:
(A) it is a branch of the internal carotid artery
(B) a haemorrhage from the middle meningeal artery results in a subdural bleed
(C) the middle meningeal artery supplies blood to the temporal lobes of the brain
(D) the middle meningeal artery ascends through the foramen spinosum
(E) the middle meningeal artery is a 'nutrient artery' to bone forming the vault of the skull

A___ B___ C___ D___ E___

10. Concerning the arteries that supply blood to the brain:
(A) branches of the basilar artery supply the pons and cerebellum
(B) the internal carotid artery lies lateral to the optic chiasma
(C) the circle of Willis lies on the basioccipital bone
(D) the anterior cerebral arteries ascend between the two frontal lobes of the brain
(E) the middle cerebral arteries supply the internal capsule

A___ B___ C___ D___ E___

11. The internal carotid artery:

(A) enters the skull through a foramen which also conducts the IXth, Xth and XIth cranial nerves
(B) divides into the anterior and middle cerebral arteries
(C) gives off the ophthalmic artery
(D) is accompanied within the skull by sympathetic nerve fibres
(E) travels through the substance of the petrous temporal bone

A ____ B ____ C ____ D ____ E ____

12. The oculomotor nerve:

(A) supplies the superior oblique muscle
(B) may be found in the lateral wall of the cavernous sinus
(C) enters the orbit through the optic canal
(D) supplies the dilator pupillae muscle
(E) carries parasympathetic fibres

A ____ B ____ C ____ D ____ E ____

13. Bones forming the medial wall of the orbital cavity include:

(A) the ethmoid
(B) the lacrimal
(C) the maxilla
(D) the sphenoid
(E) the nasal

A ____ B ____ C ____ D ____ E ____

14. The abducent nerve:

(A) supplies the levator palpebrae superioris
(B) carries fibres that supply the ciliary muscle
(C) carries parasympathetic fibres to the dilator pupillae
(D) enters the orbit through the superior orbital fissure
(E) supplies the lateral rectus muscle

A ____ B ____ C ____ D ____ E ____

15. The nasociliary nerve:

(A) is a branch of the ophthalmic division of the Vth cranial nerve
(B) enters the orbit through the optic foramen
(C) supplies some of the skin on the bridge of the nose
(D) supplies some of the mucous membrane within the nose
(E) has branches called the short ciliary nerves

A ____ B ____ C ____ D ____ E ____

16. The ciliary ganglion:

(A) is a sensory ganglion
(B) receives parasympathetic fibres from the IIIrd cranial nerve
(C) relays sympathetic fibres to the ciliary muscle
(D) has sympathetic fibres from the internal carotid plexus running through it
(E) has sensory fibres from the eyeball destined for the nasociliary nerve running through it

A ____ B ____ C ____ D ____ E ____

17. Interruption of impulses in the left cervical sympathetic trunk may result in:

(A) the pupil of the left eye being constricted
(B) the skin of the left cheek being flushed
(C) a hot dry face on the left and skin that does not sweat
(D) reduced salivary secretion being from the left parotid
(E) the upper left eyelid drooping

A ____ B ____ C ____ D ____ E ____

18. The trochlear nerve (IV):

(A) arises from the posterior aspect of the brain stem
(B) carries parasympathetic fibres
(C) innervates the lateral rectus muscle
(D) passes within the tendinous ring as it enters the orbit
(E) runs in the lateral wall of the cavernous sinus for part of its course

A ____ B ____ C ____ D ____ E ____

19. The levator palpebrae superioris:

(A) is innervated by the oculomotor nerve (III)
(B) is innervated by sympathetic nerve fibres
(C) has the frontal nerve lying above it
(D) causes drooping of the upper eyelid when it contracts
(E) inserts partly into the upper tarsal plate

A ____ B ____ C ____ D ____ E ____

20. Concerning the superior oblique muscle of the eye:

(A) it arises from the floor of the orbit on the medial side
(B) it inserts into the eyeball in front of the coronal equator
(C) when paralysed, the subject is unable to look downwards with an adducted eye
(D) it is supplied by the abducens nerve (VI)
(E) its action is normally to elevate the eye

A ____ B ____ C ____ D ____ E ____

21. The external acoustic meatus:
(A) has a sensory supply from the vagus nerve (X)
(B) has a sensory supply from the trigeminal nerve (V)
(C) can be straightened by pulling the lobule of the auricle downwards and forwards
(D) is cartilaginous for the whole of its length
(E) is approximately the same length in infants and adults

A____ B____ C____ D____ E____

22. In the middle ear:
(A) the tensor tympani is supplied by the facial nerve (VII)
(B) the ossicles are *all* united to each other by means of synovial joints
(C) the chorda tympani crosses the inner surface of the tympanic membrane
(D) the base, or footplate, of the stapes fits into the fenestra cochleae (round window)
(E) the auditory tube opens into the anterior wall of the middle ear cavity

A____ B____ C____ D____ E____

23. The facial nerve (VII):
(A) leaves the posterior cranial fossa via the internal acoustic meatus
(B) has an autonomic ganglion called the geniculate ganglion within the internal acoustic meatus
(C) passes through the stapes in company with the stapedial artery
(D) gives off the chorda tympani just below the level of the stylomastoid foramen in the parotid gland
(E) supplies both the tensor tympani and the tensor palati muscles

A____ B____ C____ D____ E____

24. The cochlea:
(A) has a basal turn that creates a promontory on the medial wall of the middle ear cavity
(B) contains cell bodies of the cochlear part of the VIIIth nerve in the modiolus
(C) has perilymph and endolymph in communication with each other at the helicotrema
(D) contains some hair cells sensitive to the pull of gravity
(E) has a fibrogelatinous tectorial membrane within the cochlear duct

A____ B____ C____ D____ E____

25. Concerning the vestibular apparatus:
(A) the membranous labyrinth is surrounded by perilymph
(B) the anterior (or superior) semicircular canal raises an arcuate eminence on the posterior surface of the petrous temporal bone
(C) hair cells of the maculae of the utricle and saccule are sensitive to the pull of gravity
(D) endolymph is secreted in the ampullae of the semicircular canals
(E) the endolymphatic duct opens into the jugular foramen.

A____ B____ C____ D____ E____

Answers to Multiple Choice Questions

1. A F	B T	C T	D T	E F	10. A T	B T	C F	D T	E T	19. A T	B T	C T	D F	E T
2. A T	B T	C F	D T	E F	11. A F	B T	C T	D T	E T	20. A F	B F	C T	D F	E F
3. A T	B T	C F	D T	E T	12. A F	B T	C F	D F	E T	21. A T	B T	C F	D F	E F
4. A F	B T	C F	D F	E T	13. A T	B T	C T	D T	E F	22. A F	B T	C T	D F	E T
5. A F	B T	C T	D F	E T	14. A F	B F	C F	D T	E T	23. A T	B F	C F	D F	E F
6. A T	B F	C F	D F	E T	15. A T	B F	C T	D T	E T	24. A T	B T	C F	D F	E T
7. A T	B F	C T	D T	E F	16. A F	B T	C F	D T	E T	25. A T	B F	C T	D F	E F
8. A T	B T	C F	D T	E F	17. A T	B T	C T	D F	E T					
9. A T	B F	C F	D T	E T	18. A T	B F	C F	D F	E T					

THE NECK, PHARYNX AND LARYNX

chapter

5

Neurovascular Structures in the Neck

Basic topography of the neck

The neck can essentially be thought of as a tube through which structures travel between the head and the trunk. The upper parts of the respiratory and digestive passageways both pass through the neck. Arterial blood courses upwards through arteries going to the head and neck, and venous blood returns to the heart in the opposite direction through veins. Several cranial nerves which leave the brain pass through foramina in the base of the skull, and then also run down through the neck.

The neck needs a strong musculoskeletal framework but at the same time it must be mobile. The seven cervical vertebrae fulfil both these functions: stability and mobility. As elsewhere in the vertebral column, pairs of spinal nerves leave through the intervertebral foramina. Surprisingly, though, there are *eight* pairs of cervical spinal nerves and not seven. This is because the first of these leaves the column *above* the first cervical vertebra. The first four pairs of these mixed nerves supply several neck muscles and are involved in cutaneous sensation of the neck. The lower pairs of spinal nerves join the brachial plexus and run into the axilla and onwards to supply the upper limb.

The cervical vertebral column is surrounded and protected by muscles. Posteriorly there is a thick extensor mass. The extensor muscle mass must be especially powerful because the head falls forwards on to the chest at rest in the upright position. A strong extensor muscle group maintains the upright position of the head (Fig. 5.1).

By the same token the flexor muscles in front of the column, the prevertebral muscles, are rather weak as in the upright position they are aided by gravity. The cervical column also gives rise to muscles that suspend the scapula on the back of the rib cage and to another set of muscles which run down to the first two ribs at the thoracic inlet (the **scalene muscles**). Each of these muscle groups that surround the cervical vertebral column is covered with fascia, which is especially well defined over the prevertebral muscles where it is called **prevertebral fascia**. It is also thick in the midline posteriorly between the extensor muscles, where it is called the **ligamentum nuchae**.

Clearly, from what we have said, we can identify two major compartments in the neck. The **anterior compartment** transmits the upper parts of the respiratory and digestive tracts (the trachea and oesophagus) as well as many neurovascular structures. The **posterior compartment** consists of the cervical vertebral column and its surrounding musculature. Both the anterior and posterior compartments are enclosed on the outside by a sheath of **investing**, or **deep cervical fascia**, that encircles the neck like a stocking (Fig. 5.1). Neurovascular structures and lymph nodes lie on either side of the structures in the anterior compartment. An endocrine gland, the **thyroid**, straddles these structures across the root of the neck.

A good way to study the topography of the neck is to start with the major vessels that run on the sides of the anterior compartment and then add to these the nerves that run with them. Following this we can describe the thyroid gland in the context of these structures and then go on to describe the pharynx and larynx in more detail.

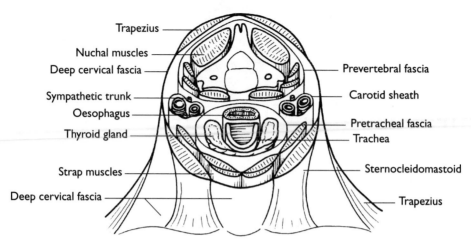

Figure 5.1   In cross-section, the cervical vertebral column of the neck can be seen to be surrounded by nuchal and prevertebral muscles, enveloped by prevertebral fascia. In front of this the oesophagus, trachea and thyroid gland are also surrounded by fascia. Great vessels and nerves lie to the side of this compartment in a loose carotid sheath. The whole of the neck itself is enveloped by deep cervical investing fascia, which encapsulates the sternocleidomastoid and trapezius muscles. (After Green JH and Silver PHS (1981) *An Introduction to Human Anatomy.* New York: Oxford Medical Publications.)

Neurovascular structures in the neck

Arteries, veins and nerves all pass through the neck; arteries ascend from the thorax and veins descend from both the head and neck. Some cranial nerves descend through the neck for a short distance but other nerves travel down the neck and into the thorax and beyond. Clearly, the skull base must be full of holes to allow things in and out of the cranial cavity.

We have already studied some of the foramina in the cranial base in Chapter 1. We now need to look at the cranial base again and take more note of the foramina through which important nerves and vessels pass (Fig. 5.2). Identify these foramina by name from the front to the back and take note of their size and shape. The **foramen ovale** is first; immediately behind is a smaller **foramen spinosum**. Further back is the neat round entrance to the **carotid canal** and then the more irregular outline of the **jugular foramen**, positioned between the temporal and occipital bones. The **stylomastoid foramen** lies between the styloid and mastoid processes. Finally, in line with the first cervical vertebra in the base of the skull, just above the occipital condyle, is the **anterior condylar foramen** or **hypoglossal canal**.

At the root of the neck there is only one hole. This is the superior aperture of the thorax or the **thoracic inlet**. Its boundaries are the first thoracic vertebra,

the two first ribs and the manubrium. Through this aperture the airway and oesophagus, as well as vessels and nerves, pass between the thorax and the neck.

Arteries pass into the right and left sides of the neck from the aorta. Two of these branches were identified in the thorax as the **brachiocephalic artery** on the right and the **common carotid artery** on the left. The brachiocephalic artery divides before ascending through the superior aperture of the thorax, and one of its divisions is the right **common carotid**

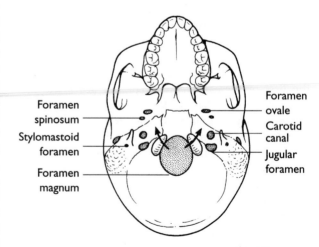

Figure 5.2   Nerves and vessels pass through foramina in the cranial base as they course between the neck and intracranial region. Observe their shape and size, and also take note of which lie most anteriorly and which most posteriorly. Arrows indicate the path of the hypoglossal canals.

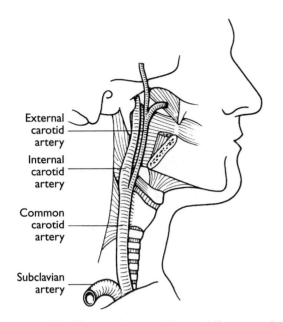

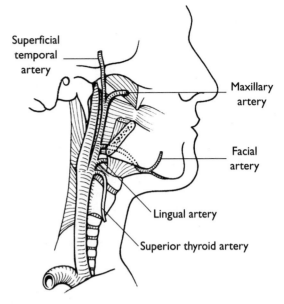

Figure 5.3 The common carotid artery bifurcates at the level of the upper border of the thyroid cartilage. The internal carotid artery continues upwards towards the carotid canal in the temporal bone. It has no branches in the neck. The external carotid artery supplies blood to structures of the neck and face.

Figure 5.4 The superior thyroid, facial and lingual arteries are major branches of the external carotid artery. The maxillary and superficial temporal arteries are the two terminal branches of the external carotid artery.

artery. Both right and left common carotids ascend the neck on the side of the midline tubes (Fig. 5.3). On reaching the level of the upper border of the thyroid cartilage each common carotid artery bifurcates into an **internal** and **external carotid artery**. The internal carotid artery is destined to supply much of the brain, and gives *no* branches in the neck during its ascent to the base of the skull. It enters the cranial cavity by passing through the carotid canal and eventually emerges close to the pituitary fossa. The external carotid artery supplies much of the neck, face, head and scalp. It therefore has several important branches. The resulting **carotid tree** can be superimposed on to the side view of the midline tubes of the neck.

Identify the important branches of the external carotid artery (Fig. 5.4). They spring from the artery at various levels. The bifurcation of the common carotid takes place at the upper border of the thyroid cartilage, a landmark that is easily palpated in a living subject. It is at this level also that the **superior thyroid artery** arises. The hyoid bone is the next landmark. This is palpable in the neck just above the thyroid cartilage, and at this level an artery to the tongue arises, the **lingual artery**. The **facial artery** arises just above the lingual artery, but here the mandible, or lower jaw, overlaps the carotid tree, and to reach the facial region the artery has to curl around the lower border of the mandible. In this position it may be felt pulsing in a living subject.

The remainder of the external carotid artery continues upwards, but to expose it the side of the mandible needs to be removed. Here in this deep part of the neck, deep to the mandible and within the substance of the parotid salivary gland, the external carotid artery divides into its two terminal branches. The **superficial temporal** branch curls behind the neck of the mandible to reach the superficial tissues of the temple and scalp. The other terminal branch, the **maxillary artery**, passes inwards towards the midline and towards its partner on the other side. On its way it supplies the upper jaw and the back of the nose and upper part of the pharynx. The external carotid artery has several other branches but these are less important.

The carotid system is not, however, the only arterial supply to the the neck. The arteries carrying blood from the aorta to the upper limbs also cross the root of the neck and help to supply some structures in the head and neck through several important branches. These arteries destined for the arms are the right and left **subclavian arteries**.

The subclavian artery

The branches of the subclavian arteries are best seen from the front at the root of the neck (Fig. 5.5). As we saw earlier, one of the branches of the subclavian artery, the **vertebral artery**, supplies part of the brain. From its origin it runs to the vertebral column in the neck and is soon lost from view as it climbs upwards through a series of foramina in the transverse processes of the cervical vertebrae. In this way it eventually reaches the cranial cavity and enters it through the foramen magnum to supply the brain. The **costocervical trunk** arises from the subclavian artery and gives a branch that supplies the deep muscles in the back of the neck and another that supplies the upper two intercostal spaces.

The **internal thoracic artery** is a branch of the subclavian artery which supplies the upper intercostal spaces and some of the small muscles of the neck. It descends into the thorax to supply the thoracic wall. The **thyrocervical trunk**, a short thick branch, divides into the **inferior thyroid artery** for the supply of the thyroid gland and two further branches which pass back to the shoulder region and to the scapular muscles (Fig. 5.6). The most important branches of the subclavian artery for you to remember are the inferior thyroid artery, the vertebral artery and the internal thoracic artery. The inferior thyroid artery is important because of

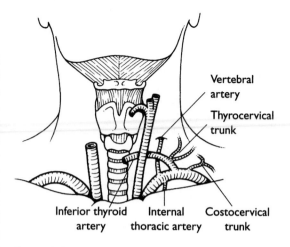

Figure 5.6 The inferior thyroid artery arises from the thyrocervical trunk. It passes posteriorly, behind the common carotid artery, to reach the thyroid gland.

its close relationship to a nerve that runs to the larynx, and the vertebral artery because it supplies the brain.

Venous drainage of the head and neck

The internal jugular vein, after draining blood from the brain via the intracranial venous sinuses, enters

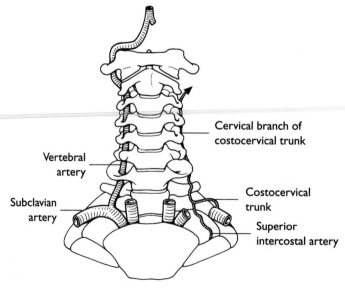

Figure 5.5 The vertebral artery arises from the subclavian artery in the root of the neck. It ascends through the foramina transversaria of the cervical vertebrae and passes through the foramen magnum to form the basilar artery with the contralateral vertebral artery. The costocervical trunk gives branches to the deep structures of the neck and to the superior intercostal spaces.

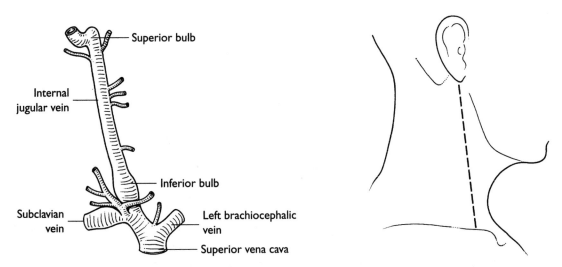

Figure 5.7 (a) The internal jugular vein arises at the superior jugular bulb in the jugular foramen. It receives tributaries from structures in the neck including the thyroid gland. The inferior jugular bulb has valves just above it which prevent back flow of blood when the intrathoracic pressure is raised (as when lifting or straining). (b) The surface marking of the internal jugular vein runs deep to a line connecting a point overlying the arch of the atlas above (between the tragus of the ear and the mastoid process) and the sternoclavicular joint below.

the neck through the jugular foramen. It first follows the internal and then the common carotid arteries downwards to the root of the neck, running at all times lateral to them. On the way down, the internal jugular veins receive superficial venous drainage from the scalp, face and neck (Fig. 5.7). They also receive the deep venous tributaries of the neck. At the root of the neck each internal jugular vein joins with the subclavian vein to form a brachiocephalic vein. The two brachiocephalic veins run down behind the manubrium and join to form the superior vena cava.

The surface marking of the internal jugular vein is important since it is one vein used to pass catheters into the heart. The jugular foramen lies in front of the arch of the atlas at the skull base. This point is midway between the mastoid process and the tragus of the auricle when the face is turned to the side. The vein then passes directly towards and then behind the sternoclavicular joint (Fig. 5.7). It lies beneath the cleft between the two heads of sternocleidomastoid here.

Lying along the vascular pathways in the neck are lymphatics. At various intervals along them are lymph nodes, which are especially numerous beside the internal jugular vein. The pattern and distribution of lymph nodes in the neck will be described later in more detail in Chapter 8.

Cranial nerves in the neck

Several cranial nerves enter the neck through foramina in the base of the skull. The Vth cranial nerve or **trigeminal nerve** has three divisions. One of these, the mandibular division (Viii), passes down towards the mouth and mandible. The VIIth cranial nerve, the **facial nerve**, is running to the muscles of facial expression. Other cranial nerves also leave the cranial base and travel in the neck for some way. These include the IXth (or **glossopharyngeal nerve**), Xth (**vagus**), XIth (**accessory**) and XIIth (**hypoglossal**), and each requires thoughtful study.

The mandibular division of the Vth nerve and the VIIth cranial nerve can be put in context now and then studied in detail later since they are nerves that belong to the mouth and face. The mandibular nerve (Viii) leaves the cranial cavity through the foramen ovale and the facial nerve (VII) through the **stylo-mastoid foramen**. (As its name implies, you will find this foramen between the styloid and mastoid processes on the skull base.) The mandibular nerve then runs deep to the mandible and the facial nerve superficial to the mandible. The former innervates structures in the mouth and the latter the muscles of the face.

Cranial nerves IX, X and XI emerge together

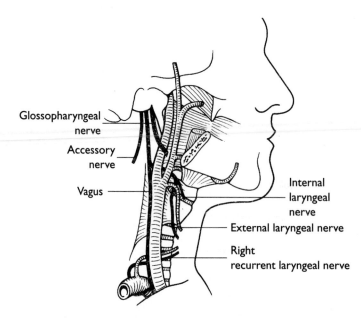

Figure 5.8 The relationship between the IXth, Xth and XIth cranial nerves in the neck and the carotid tree.

through the jugular foramen. Cranial nerve XII emerges from the posterior cranial fossa through the anterior condylar foramen or hypoglossal canal. In this way all of these nerves are at first arranged quite close to the internal carotid artery and internal jugular vein. However, when these nerves are traced down the neck they spread out to reach their destinations. In so doing they come into important relationships with both the carotid tree and its branches and the subclavian artery and its branches. In this way they form so called neurovascular bundles. Figure 5.8 shows the topography of some of these neurovascular bundles. The glossopharyngeal nerve (IX) runs to the pharynx and the posterior part of the tongue, and therefore aims for the wall of the pharynx. The vagus nerve (X) follows closely the path of the internal and common carotid arteries downwards through the neck. It then runs in front of the subclavian artery to leave the neck through the superior aperture of the thorax. Two of its branches are of particular importance in the neck since they supply the larynx. These laryngeal branches aim for the upper and lower boundaries of the larynx respectively. The accessory nerve (XI) passes downwards and backwards, and enters two large muscles, the **sternocleidomastoid** and **trapezius** muscles, which we will study later on. The hypoglossal nerve (XII) supplies the musculature of the tongue and so passes deep to the muscles of the floor of the mouth.

Look at these important cranial nerves and at the branches of the external carotid and subclavian arteries and notice how each nerve runs with a branch of either one or other artery. After leaving the skull through the jugular foramen the glossopharyngeal nerve passes *between* the internal and external carotid arteries to reach its destination. It arrives at the upper border of the **middle constrictor muscle** of the pharynx where it contributes to the sensory nerve supply of the pharynx. It then runs just lateral to the palatine tonsil in the wall of the oropharynx and runs to supply the posterior one-third of the tongue. A fine filamentous branch of the glossopharyngeal nerve runs down to the bifurcation of the carotids. Here it supplies specialized tissue in the **carotid sinus** and the **carotid body**. These structures help to monitor and regulate blood pressure and blood gas concentrations.

The vagus nerve (X) also enters the neck through the jugular foramen. It closely follows the course of the internal and common carotid arteries and internal jugular vein. It therefore contributes to a great neurovascular bundle with these vessels. The bundle is loosely bound by connective tissue and is known as the **carotid sheath**. The vagus nerve runs down the sheath and eventually over the front of the subclavian artery to enter the thorax. Soon after leaving the skull the vagus gives off a **pharyngeal branch**. These fibres form a meshwork on the surface of the pharyngeal muscles, and carry motor fibres to the pharynx and palate.

The uppermost branch to the larynx is the **superior laryngeal nerve**. This divides to give a *sensory* branch (the **internal laryngeal nerve**), which enters the larynx by piercing a membrane, and a *motor* branch (the **external laryngeal nerve**), destined to supply one important muscle on the surface of the larynx. For part of its course the superior laryngeal nerve follows the superior thyroid artery, so forming a neurovascular bundle.

The lower branch on the right (Fig. 5.8) is the **right recurrent laryngeal nerve**. This branch hooks around the right subclavian artery and ascends with the inferior thyroid artery, so forming another important neurovascular bundle. This nerve enters the larynx to supply the remainder of the laryngeal musculature. The **left recurrent laryngeal nerve** arises in the thorax and hooks around the arch of the aorta before ascending into the neck. Its terminal part has the same relationship to the inferior thyroid artery as the right recurrent laryngeal nerve.

The accessory nerve (XI) arises in two parts. Some fibres arise from the brain just below the vagus (X) and others arise from the upper part of the spinal cord. The former group of fibres is called the **cranial root** and the latter the **spinal root** of the accessory nerve. The two roots join and converge on the vagus nerve just before the Xth and XIth nerves leave the skull. When they have passed through the jugular foramen they separate again and the cranial fibres of the accessory join the vagus and the spinal fibres of the accessory travel on as a separate nerve.

Before we leave our description of the vagus nerve it is essential for you to understand that the 'vagus nerve' entering the neck is actually a mixture of **vagoaccessory** fibres (a mixture of vagal fibres and *cranial* accessory fibres, in fact). By the same reasoning, the 'accessory nerve' in the neck is more accurately the spinal part of the accessory nerve. The vagoaccessory mixture supplies motor fibres to the muscles of the pharynx through the **pharyngeal branch** of the vagus. This motor pharyngeal complex, together with some sensory fibres from the glossopharyngeal nerve IX (and a few sympathetic fibres), forms a meshwork of nerve fibres on the pharyngeal wall called the **pharyngeal plexus**. The plexus supplies motor and sensory nerve fibres to the pharynx and motor supply to the muscles of the soft palate (except, as we will discover later, tensor palati). The laryngeal nerves also contain a mixture of true vagal and

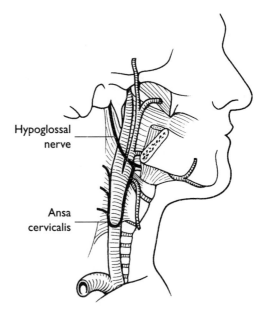

Figure 5.9 The relationship between the XIIth cranial nerve in the neck and the carotid tree.

cranial accessory fibres. However, by the time the main vagal trunks have reached the thorax, en route to the abdomen, all the cranial accessory fibres have been used up, together with some vagal fibres, in supplying the muscles of the pharynx, larynx and soft palate. What we see in the thorax and abdomen are therefore 'true' vagal fibres and not a mixture as in the neck.

The hypoglossal nerve (XII) is for the most part a nerve of transit in the neck. It supplies almost all of the tongue muscles and therefore aims for the lingual artery, travelling with it as a neurovascular bundle (Fig. 5.9). It begins as the most medially placed cranial nerve as it exits the cranial cavity through the hypoglossal canal. But from this position it takes a wide embracing course around both the internal and external carotids and also outside the loop of the lingual artery. Although it is a nerve of transit it does carry some fibres that 'hitch-hike' along it for a short distance. A few fibres from the first cervical ventral ramus run with the hypoglossal nerve close to the skull base. These fibres 'hitch-hike' along it for a while and then leave it as a slender filament called the **superior root of the ansa cervicalis**. Fibres from the 2nd and 3rd cervical ventral rami form the so-called **inferior root of the ansa cervicalis**. The two join to form a delicate U-shaped loop on the common carotid artery and internal jugular vein

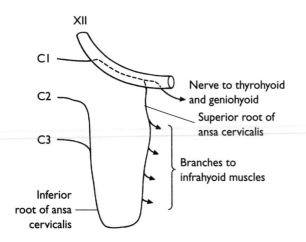

Figure 5.10   Nerve fibres from the ventral ramus of CI run in company with the hypoglossal nerve. Some run on to supply the geniohyoid and thyrohyoid muscles. Other fibres drop inferiorly as the superior root of the ansa cervicalis and join with fibres of C2 and C3, which form the inferior root of the ansa cervicalis. Branches from the ansa supply the infrahyoid strap muscles.

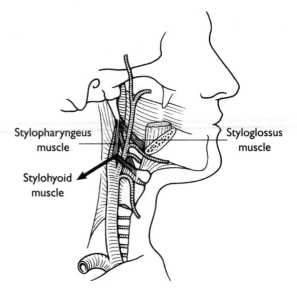

Figure 5.11   The relationship of the three styloid muscles, stylohyoid, styloglossus and stylopharyngeus, to the carotid tree.

The thyroid gland

The thyroid gland is an important endocrine gland composed of two **lateral lobes**. It lies on each side of the larynx and upper tracheal cartilages and overlaps the carotid sheaths. The two lobes are joined in front

(Fig. 5.10). These cervical nerve fibres are destined to supply some of the strap-like muscles at the front of the neck.

Three small **styloid muscles** weave through the carotid tree from the bony styloid process on the base of the skull and complete our picture of the deep structures at the side of the neck (Fig. 5.11). The **styloglossus**, destined for the tongue, is a deep muscle and will be discussed later since it belongs functionally to the mouth. The **stylopharyngeus** passes with the glossopharyngeal nerve (IX). First it passes between the external and internal carotid arteries and then over the upper border of the middle constrictor. It is a longitudinal muscle of the pharynx. The **stylohyoid** muscle is more superficial, and runs around the carotid tree (just like the hypoglossal nerve) to insert into the hyoid bone.

At this point you should be aware that there are a few important smaller branches of the external carotid artery (Fig. 5.12). The **ascending pharyngeal** artery arises opposite the superior thyroid artery and supplies blood to the pharyngeal wall. The **occipital artery** arises opposite the facial artery and passes to the back of the neck, deep to the sternocleidomastoid muscle. The **posterior auricular** branch runs out of the parotid gland near the neck of the mandible and supplies adjacent parts of the gland as well as skin and muscles here.

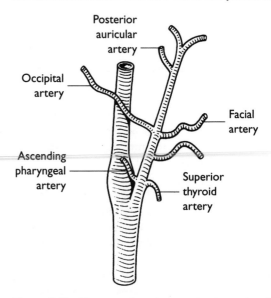

Figure 5.12   The ascending pharyngeal artery arises from the posterior aspect of the external carotid artery at the level of origin of the superior thyroid artery. The occipital artery arises opposite the facial artery and the posterior auricular artery is given off in the parotid gland prior to the terminal division of the external carotid.

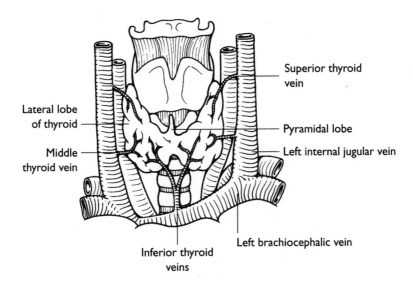

Lateral lobe of thyroid

Middle thyroid vein

Superior thyroid vein

Pyramidal lobe

Left internal jugular vein

Inferior thyroid veins

Left brachiocephalic vein

Figure 5.13 The isthmus of the thyroid gland lies in the midline and the lateral lobes of the thyroid either side of the trachea, cricoid and thyroid cartilages. The pyramidal lobe, when present, is drawn out along the embryological path of migration of the thyroid gland. Usually there are three groups of veins draining the thyroid gland.

of the trachea by an **isthmus** of thyroid tissue (Fig. 5.13). Each lobe is conical in shape. The lower part of the medial surface is moulded against the trachea and oesophagus, where the recurrent laryngeal nerve lies in the groove between these structures. The upper part of the medial surface is placed against the **cricoid** and **thyroid** cartilages, and it comes into relationship with the motor branch of the superior laryngeal nerve, the external laryngeal branch.

Two small **parathyroid glands** are embedded in the posterior surface of each lobe. These ductless endocrine glands are concerned with the maintenance of body calcium levels (Fig. 5.14). The **superior parathyroid** is relatively constant in position, lying in the middle of the posterior surface of the lobe. The **inferior parathyroid**, however, lies near the **inferior pole** of the lobe or even amongst the structures below the lobe. The reason for its variable level is that the inferior parathyroid develops with the **thymus gland**. This latter gland descends into the anterior mediastinum of the thorax during development and drags the inferior parathyroid with it. It can be imagined that the final resting place for this parathyroid may be anywhere along the path of descent.

The isthmus of the thyroid lies over the second, third and fourth tracheal rings, and joins the two lateral lobes. Often, a tongue of glandular thyroid tissue springs from the upper border of the isthmus and extends upwards towards the hyoid bone. This is called the **pyramidal lobe** of the thyroid gland. Indeed,

it can even be attached to the hyoid by a small muscular slip known as the **levator glandulae thyroideae**. Occasionally, the muscle is represented only by a strand of fibrous tissue.

The thyroid gland develops from the floor of the embryological pharynx. Its site of origin can be seen in the adult near the back of the tongue as a small depression, the **foramen caecum**. From this position the cells of the future gland multiply and descend into the neck, passing in front of the hyoid bone, looping up *behind* the bone and finally descending to reach their adult position (Fig. 5.15). Sometimes small clusters of glandular thyroid tissue are found along this pathway in the adult and may present as midine swellings in the neck. If glandular thyroid tissue develops in the region of the foramen caecum on the tongue it is called a **lingual thyroid**. The occasional fibrous slip or pyramidal lobe uniting the isthmus to the hyoid is also a developmental remnant (Fig. 5.13).

The lobes and isthmus of the thyroid are enclosed in a sheath of fascia which is part of the sheet of fascia called the **pretracheal fascia**. This is attached to the thyroid cartilage and to the cricoid cartilage of the larynx. At the sides it blends with the fascia of the carotid sheaths. Because of the attachment of the fascia to the thyroid and cricoid cartilages, the thyroid gland moves up and down with the larynx during swallowing. Below, the pretracheal fascia blends with the fascia over the arch of the aorta.

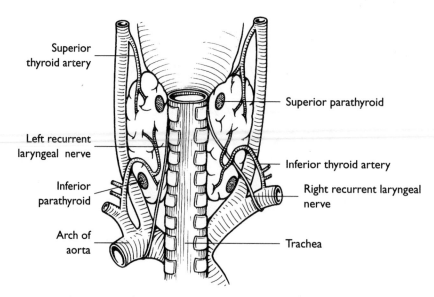

Figure 5.14 The trachea, thyroid and parathyroid glands seen from behind. Notice the close relationship between the inferior thyroid arteries and the recurrent laryngeal nerves. (After Hollinshead WH (1982) *Anatomy for Surgeons*, Philadelphia: Harper and Row.)

We identified the superior thyroid artery as one of the branches of the external carotid. In its descent it runs in close relationship with the external laryngeal

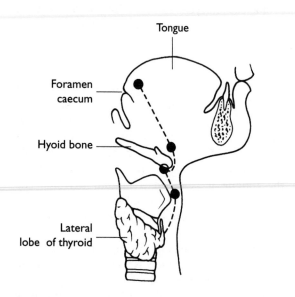

Figure 5.15 The embryological origin of the thyroid gland is represented by the foramen caecum of the tongue. The dotted line represents the path of migration of the thyroid gland during development to its adult position overlying the trachea. Remnants of thyroid tissue or cysts may occur and present as midline swellings in the neck at any position along this path of migration. (After Basmajian JV and Slonecker CE (1989) *Grant's Method of Anatomy*, 11th edn. Baltimore: Williams and Wilkins.)

nerve. The inferior thyroid artery was identified as a branch of the subclavian artery. This artery passes deeply, *behind* the carotid sheath towards the gland, and then divides here. Its branches lie in close relationship to the recurrent laryngeal nerve (Fig. 5.15). Thus, in thyroid surgery care must be taken to preserve the external laryngeal nerve when ligating the superior thyroid artery and to preserve the recurrent laryngeal nerve when ligating the inferior thyroid artery. Occasionally, a small artery, called the **thyroid ima**, arises directly from the arch of the aorta, brachiocephalic artery or left common carotid artery and ascends over the front of the trachea to supply the isthmus of the thyroid gland. All of these thyroid arteries anastomose freely on the surface of the gland in the space between the pretracheal fascial sheath and the true capsule of the gland (a layer of condensed tissue on the outer surface of the gland).

Blood is collected into a venous network which is also found on the surface of the gland. From here it drains through three pairs of veins. The **superior** and **middle thyroid veins** enter the internal jugular vein. The **inferior thyroid vein** or veins descend through the superior aperture of the thorax to drain into the brachiocephalic veins behind the manubrium.

Lymphatics around the thyroid follow vascular patterns and drain to nodes around the carotid sheath and the root of the neck. A few also drain into upper mediastinal nodes in the thorax.

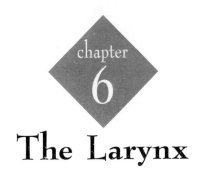

The Larynx

The larynx is a valve that protects the entrance to the airway or tracheobronchial tree. It is also involved in the production of speech sounds and in phonation in humans. If its protective role is ineffective, laryngeal incompetence can lead to food and fluid being aspirated into the trachea. The larynx is composed of four major cartilages united by mobile synovial joints. Ligaments and membranes also fill in the gaps between them. The larynx has outer and inner walls which rise from a circular base (the cricoid ring) rather like two flower pots, one placed inside the other.

The cartilages and membranes of the larynx

The **thyroid cartilage** with the **thyrohyoid membrane**, together with the **cricoid cartilage** and the **cricothyroid membrane**, form the outer wall (Fig. 6.1). The thyroid cartilage is the largest cartilage and consists of two **laminae** which meet in the midline at an angle. The thyroid cartilage projects as a **laryngeal prominence**, and this may be seen and palpated in the midline of the neck (especially in men because the angle between the laminae becomes more acute at puberty). A **superior thyroid notch** can be palpated between the two laminae above the laryngeal prominence. The posterior border of each thyroid cartilage is extended above and below as slender superior and inferior **horns** (or **cornua**).

The cricoid cartilage is the shape of a signet ring, the narrow part of the ring lying in front and the thick section behind. The front of the cricoid may be palpated in the neck below the thyroid cartilage. The inferior cornu of each thyroid lamina articulates with a facet on the side of the cricoid at a synovial articulation. The outer wall of the larynx is completed by several membranes. The upper border of each lamina of the thyroid cartilage gives attachment to the thyrohyoid membrane. This stretches upwards to gain attachment to the inner border of the **hyoid bone** in the floor of the mouth. The lower border of the thyroid cartilage is attached to the cricoid in the midline by the strong **cricothyroid ligament**, and, below, the cricoid is attached to the uppermost ring of the trachea by the **cricotracheal ligament**.

The inner wall of the larynx is composed of membrane, muscles, the **arytenoid cartilages** posteriorly and the **epiglottis** above. The structure of the inner wall is best appreciated by removing one thyroid lamina (Fig. 6.2). The leaf-like epiglottis is attached by a ligament to the inner surface of the angle of the thyroid laminae. It projects upwards behind the thyrohyoid membrane, hyoid bone and tongue. Paired arytenoid cartilages sit on the upper border of the lamina of the cricoid. Each arytenoid cartilage is pyramidal in shape. The joint between each arytenoid base and the cricoid is synovial. The inner wall of the larynx is completed by a membrane which extends from the sides of the epiglottis above to the arytenoids behind, and down to the lower part of the thyroid cartilage below. The part of this fibroelastic membrane between the side of the epiglottis and arytenoid is called the **quadrangular membrane**. It ends below at a sharp free border that runs between the arytenoid behind and the thyroid lamina in front. This free edge

(a)

(b)

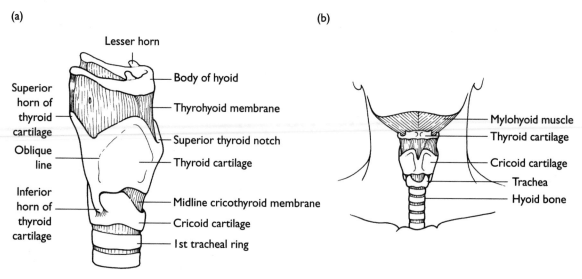

Figure 6.1 The hyoid bone, thyroid cartilage, cricoid cartilage and trachea with their associated membranes seen from the side (a) and the front (b).

is called the **vestibular ligament**. The upper part of the quadrangular membrane is far less well developed, and is replaced by muscle fibres. There is a slit-like gap below the vestibular ligament.

Beneath this slit lies the **conus elasticus** or **crico-vocal membrane**. The superficial part of the conus elasticus in the midline anteriorly is called the crico-thyroid ligament. The conus elasticus arises from the circular cricoid base and ends at an upper free border which forms the lower edge of the slit in the inner wall of the larynx. The free border of the conus elasticus is fixed at both front and back within the larynx. It runs between the **anterior process** (or **vocal process**) on the base of the arytenoid cartilage posteriorly to the midline of the two thyroid laminae anteriorly. The thickened free edge of the conus elasticus is called the **vocal ligament**. When covered with mucous membrane it is called the **vocal fold**.

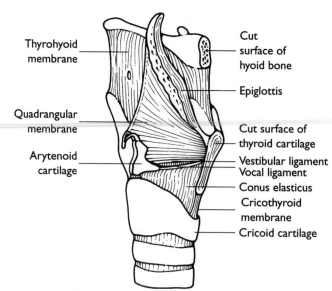

Figure 6.2 One thyroid lamina and one quadrangular membrane have been removed in this view. The conus elasticus arises from the base of the cricoid cartilage and ends above as the vocal ligament. The quadrangular membrane has a free lower border called the vestibular ligament. The vocal ligament and the quadrangular ligament run between the arytenoid cartilages and the thyroid cartilage.

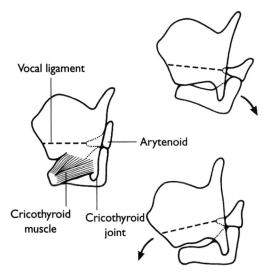

Figure 6.3 Rocking movements of the thyroid cartilage on the cricoid (or vice versa) at the cricothyroid joint tense the vocal ligament. The ligament runs from the vocal process of the arytenoid to the thyroid cartilage anteriorly.

The thyroid, cricoid and most of the arytenoid cartilages are made of hyaline cartilage. The epiglottis and apices of the arytenoids are made of elastic fibrocartilage. Two small pea-like **corniculate** and **cuneiform** cartilages are located along the upper border of the quadrangular membrane and its associated muscle.

Movements of the laryngeal cartilages

The structures involved in the production of sound and in regulation of the airway size are the **vocal ligaments**. It is therefore important to understand how movements at the cricothyroid and cricoarytenoid joints produce changes in the tension and position of these ligaments. Movement occurs at the two cricothyroid joints around a transverse axis. A movement at the cricothyroid joints which tilts the thyroid cartilage forwards will increase tension of the vocal ligaments (Fig. 6.3). A movement in the opposite direction relaxes the ligaments. Movements at the cricothyroid joints are therefore responsible for changes in *tension* in the vocal ligaments.

Movements at the cricoarytenoid joints are more complex. The cartilages may be abducted away from the laryngeal midline or adducted towards it. In other

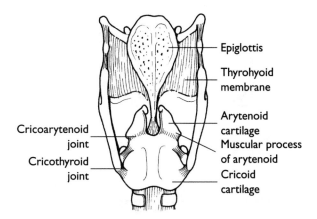

Figure 6.4 The laryngeal cartilages seen from behind. The arytenoid cartilages are pyramidal structures that articulate at cylindrically shaped synovial joints with the cricoid cartilage.

words they may slide away from or towards, each other and so take the vocal processes away from or towards the midline (Fig. 6.4). The vocal folds also move apart on deep inspiration, probably due simply to the trachea stretching downwards and drawing the mucous membrane around the laryngeal inlet with it. Thus the gap between the vocal ligaments, the **rima glottidis**, alters in both size and shape with abduction and adduction of the vocal ligaments and on deep inspiration. Figure 6.5(a) shows the arytenoids and vocal ligaments in the adducted position, with a triangular shape to the rima glottidis, while Figure 6.5(b) shows the arytenoids both widely abducted. Lateral movements of the arytenoids occur, therefore, as the size and shape of the rima glottidis varies. The cricoarytenoid joints are more than likely cylindrical in nature and also allow an anteroposterior rocking movement. When the arytenoids rock forwards they relax the vocal ligaments, whereas a backward pull increases tension in the ligaments. These movements, however, are opposed by muscles that pull in the opposite directions.

The muscles that move the laryngeal cartilages at the cricothyroid and cricoarytenoid joints are called the **intrinsic muscles** of the larynx. **Extrinsic muscles** run between the larynx and neighbouring structures and move the larynx as a whole up and down the neck. The intrinsic muscles may be divided functionally into three groups. First, there are muscles that move the epiglottis and close the laryngeal inlet; second, there are muscles responsible for abduction and adduction of the cords; and finally there are muscles that affect tension in the cords.

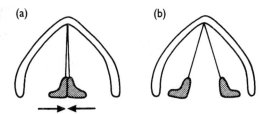

Figure 6.5 The laryngeal inlet seen from above. Medial and lateral sliding movements of the arytenoid cartilages adduct (a) and abduct (b) the vocal ligaments.

Muscles of the laryngeal inlet

There is a muscle in each aryepiglottic fold extending from the apex of the arytenoid cartilage to the side of the epiglottis. This is the **aryepiglottic muscle** (Fig. 6.6). Its fibres may be traced onwards from the posterior end of each muscle across the back of the larynx to the opposite arytenoid cartilage. These are the **oblique arytenoid muscles**. The two cross each other behind the arytenoid cartilages. The aryepiglottic muscles and the oblique arytenoids together form a **sphincter of the inlet** of the larynx. Their contraction brings the **aryepiglottic folds** together, and the epiglottis closer to the arytenoid cartilages. In addition, other muscle fibres sweep up from the inside of the thyroid cartilage into the epiglottis on each side. These are the **thyroepiglottic** muscles, whose action is to open the inlet of the larynx. Other muscle fibres in the wall of the inlet assist with this. This strong sphincteric action at the inlet can resist high intrathoracic pressures, as when coughing or lifting heavy objects.

Muscles that abduct and adduct the cords

Abduction and adduction of the vocal folds, or cords, increases and decreases the volume of air passing through the larynx. It is probably not possible to say for sure what the action of each intrinsic muscle of the larynx is in this respect since they all are likely to be active together during both abduction and adduction of the vocal folds. It is important to remember that stretching of the trachea during deep inspiration, and also activity in the sternothyroid muscle, both bring about abduction of the vocal folds, inde-

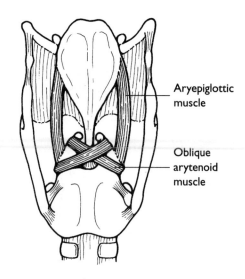

Aryepiglottic muscle

Oblique arytenoid muscle

Figure 6.6 The aryepiglottic muscles run in the upper margins of the quadrangular membranes between the epiglottis and the arytenoid cartilage, and act like a sphincter here. The oblique arytenoid muscles cross each other on the posterior aspect of the arytenoid cartilages. All these muscles have a sphincteric action around the vestibule and inlet of the larynx.

pendent of the intrinsic musculature of the larynx. Classically, only one pair of intrinsic muscles was described as abducting the vocal cords, the **posterior cricoarytenoids**. Each arises from the back of the cricoid and converges on to the **lateral angle** of the arytenoid cartilage, a point referred to as the **muscular process**. This muscle is large and fan-shaped (Fig. 6.7). Many descriptions hold that the upper fibres act by rotating the arytenoid cartilage so that its vocal process turns laterally, a movement that abducts the vocal cord. You should be aware, however, that if the cricoarytenoid joint really is cylindrical in form, this rotation would not be possible. Not all authorities accept that there is rotation of the arytenoids about a vertical axis. The most lateral fibres of the posterior cricoarytenoid are oriented in a way that could pull the arytenoid as a whole laterally, with a gliding movement at the cricoarytenoid joint. This is how many people think the vocal folds are abducted. The posterior cricoarytenoids also resist the pull of the cricothyroid muscle (see below), which acts to tense the vocal ligament. Without this resistance from behind, the arytenoid cartilages would simply fall forwards when there is strong contraction of the cricothyroid muscles.

The **lateral cricoarytenoid** muscle (Fig. 6.8) arises from the lateral side of the cricoid and runs obliquely

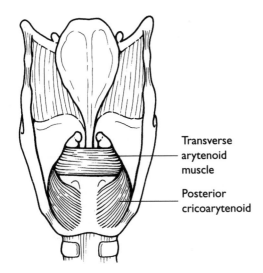

Figure 6.7 The posterior cricoarytenoid muscles sweep round from the back of the cricoid cartilage to attach to the muscular processes of the arytenoids. These muscles draw the arytenoid cartilages apart. The transverse arytenoids (together with the oblique arytenoids) pull the arytenoid cartilages together.

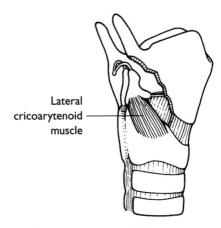

Figure 6.8 The lateral cricoarytenoid muscles also run from the cricoid to the muscular processes of each arytenoid cartilage. The muscle fibres draw the arytenoid cartilages laterally along with the fibres of posterior cricoarytenoid.

to the muscular process of the arytenoid. Again, the muscle is positioned appropriately for it to act with the posterior cricoarytenoid muscle and abduct the vocal ligaments, but it is unlikely ever to act alone in so doing.

Another muscle besides the oblique arytenoids that must act to bring the arytenoids and vocal ligaments together is the **transverse arytenoid** muscle (Fig. 6.9), which passes horizontally from one arytenoid to the other at the back of the larynx.

Muscles that tense and relax the vocal ligaments

Altering the tension of the vocal ligaments changes the pitch of the voice, and is mainly controlled by the **thyroarytenoid** and **cricothyroid muscles**. The thyroarytenoid is a complex muscle that arises from the interior midline angle of the thyroid cartilage (Fig. 6.9). It sweeps backwards to its insertion into the anterolateral surface of the arytenoid cartilage. Some fibres, however, ascend to the epiglottis and have already been described above as the thyroepiglottic muscle. This part of the muscle widens the laryngeal inlet. The main bulk of the thyroarytenoid complex, however, draws the arytenoid cartilages forwards and

relaxes the vocal ligament. A deep, triangular bundle of fibres of the thyroarytenoid complex called the **vocalis** lies close to the vocal ligament. These fibres are able selectively to separate one part of the vocal ligament while the rest remains adducted (Fig. 6.9). The vocalis muscle fibres assist in producing sounds of the highest pitch when the vocal ligaments are already maximally tensed by the cricothyroid muscle.

The cricothyroid muscles oppose the pull of the posterior cricoarytenoid muscles on the arytenoid cartilages and also the pull of the thyroarytenoids, which act to shorten the span between the thyroid cartilage and the arytenoids. The cricothyroid muscles lie on the outer surface of the larynx and produce tension in the vocal ligaments (Fig. 6.10). These muscles are particularly involved in the production of high voice tones. They act by tilting the cricoid cartilage relative to the thyroid, and vice versa, at the cricothyroid joints. The posterior cricoarytenoid muscles assist the tensing action of the cricothyroids by pulling back on the arytenoids.

The interior of the larynx

The interior of the larynx is lined with mucous membrane. This is reflected from the tongue on to the epiglottis and the mucous membrane is thrown into one **median** and two **lateral glossoepiglottic folds** in this region (Fig. 6.11). The depression on each side

(a)

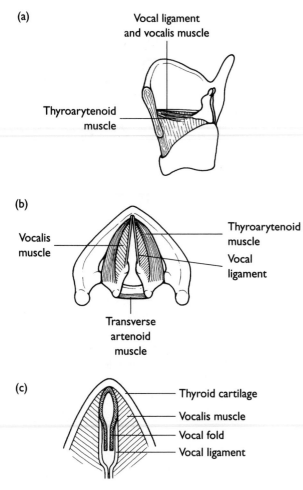

Vocal ligament
and vocalis muscle

Thyroarytenoid
muscle

(b)

Vocalis
muscle

Thyroarytenoid
muscle

Vocal
ligament

Transverse
artenoid
muscle

(c)

Thyroid cartilage

Vocalis muscle

Vocal fold

Vocal ligament

Figure 6.9   The thyroarytenoid muscles run from the thyroid cartilage to the arytenoids (a) and (b). An inner portion of this muscle, the vocalis, runs into the edge of the vocal ligament and is able to separate parts of the tensed vocal ligaments while the rest remain abducted (c). (After Hollinshead WH (1982) *Anatomy for Surgeons*, Philadelphia: Harper and Row.)

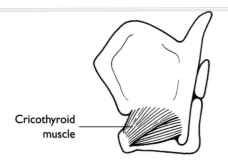

Cricothyroid
muscle

Figure 6.10   The cricothyroid muscle acts across the synovial cricothyroid joint between the lesser cornu of the thyroid cartilage and the facet for it on the cricoid cartilage. It tenses the vocal ligaments.

of the median fold is called the **vallecula**. Between the outer and inner walls of the larynx, the mucous membrane forms a **piriform recess** or **fossa** on each side (Fig. 6.12). The plane of the inlet of the larynx is almost vertical and leads into the upper part of the larynx or **vestibule**. The vestibule of the larynx extends from the inlet down to the vestibular ligaments. The gap between the two vestibular folds is called the **rima vestibuli**. Between the vestibular folds and the vocal folds there is an opening that leads into the so-called **ventricle of the larynx** (Fig. 6.12). The most anterior aspect of this recess is called the **saccule of the larynx**. The ventricle and saccule extend upwards on the outer side of the quadrangular membrane.

The laryngeal nerves

The nerve supply for the larynx comes from the vagus nerve through its superior and recurrent laryngeal branches (Fig. 6.13). The superior laryngeal nerve leaves the vagus high in the neck, and after passing deep to both carotids it divides into internal and external branches. The **internal laryngeal nerve** enters the larynx by piercing the thyrohyoid membrane and supplies sensation to the mucous membrane of the larynx above the vocal cords, which includes the piriform fossa. The nerve also supplies both surfaces of the epiglottis, the aryepiglottic fold and each vallecula. The external laryngeal branch of the superior laryngeal nerve supplies the cricothyroid muscle. In its course towards this muscle on the outside of the larynx, it is closely associated with the superior thyroid artery, and must be protected when ligating this vessel during operations on the thyroid gland.

The recurrent laryngeal nerve enters the larynx behind the cricothyroid joint. It supplies all of the intrinsic muscles of the larynx, *except* cricothyroid, and sensation to the mucous membrane below the vocal folds. Terminal branches mingle with those of the superior laryngeal nerve. The **cricopharyngeal** part of the **inferior constrictor** of the pharynx is often supplied by twigs from either the recurrent nerve or the external laryngeal nerve. During its course towards the larynx, the recurrent laryngeal nerve is closely associated with the inferior thyroid artery, and damage to the nerve is a hazard during thyroidectomy.

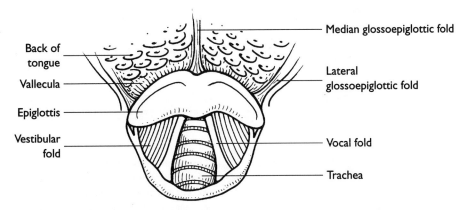

Figure 6.11 The base of the tongue and the laryngeal inlet seen from above. A median and two lateral glossoepiglottic folds run from the base of the tongue to the epiglottis. The valleculae are depressions that lie between these folds on either side of the midline.

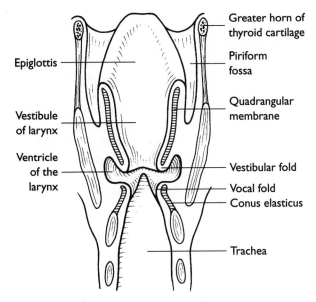

Figure 6.12 The larynx seen in longitudinal section from behind. The piriform fossae lie between the quadrangular membrane and epiglottis and the mucous membrane covering the thyroid cartilage and the hyoid bone. Between the vestibular and vocal folds there is an opening into the ventricle of the larynx. The most anterior part of this recess is called the saccule.

Lymphatic drainage of the larynx

Lymphatic drainage of the larynx becomes important in malignant disease. Lymphatics carry tumour cells first to local lymph nodes in the neck and eventually from here they spread widely throughout the body. The lymphatics of the larynx form two distinct systems, one above and the other below the vocal cords; however, anastomoses between the two systems occur in the posterior wall of the larynx. The lymphatics from the upper group pierce the thyrohyoid membrane and follow the superior laryngeal vessels. They reach the **upper deep cervical nodes**. The lower vessels pierce the cricovocal membrane and drain into **pretracheal nodes** on the cricovocal membrane and into **paratracheal nodes** along the course of the recurrent laryngeal nerve.

Applied anatomy of the larynx

A patent airway is vital for life. The most common obstruction to the airway results from food or other objects becoming lodged in the laryngeal inlet. This, together with spasm of the laryngeal muscles, occludes the airway. More often than not this sort of obstruction can be dislodged by either coughing or by a finger removing the bolus, or by sharply compressing the subject's chest from behind with tightly interlocked arms. Failure to achieve an airway by any of these simple means is serious and in an emergency situation an incision can be made through the cricothyroid membrane in the midline. This lies below the level of the vocal folds and at the entrance into the trachea. Awkward items that are usually swallowed with difficulty often tend to get stuck in the piriform fossa and sometimes need to be removed.

Anaesthetists, especially, recognize the importance of being able to identify the valleculae at the base of

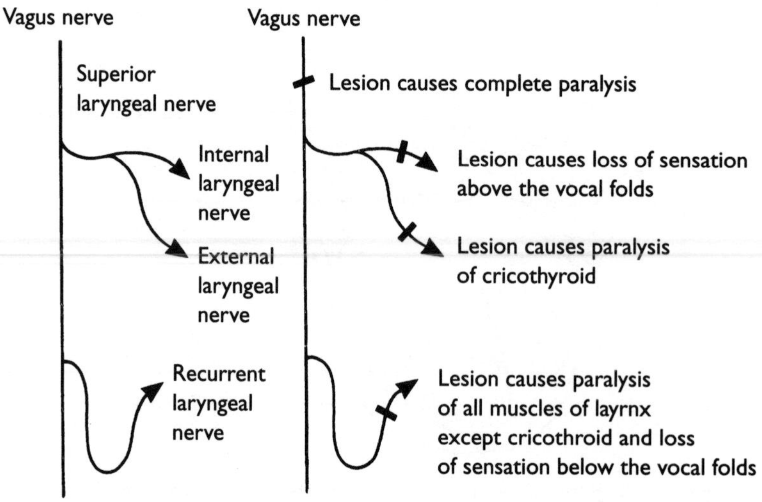

Figure 6.13 Diagramatic representation of the laryngeal branches of the vagus nerve and their motor and sensory distribution.

the tongue when intubating patients. The tip of a laryngoscope is placed in the vallecula and the base of the tongue drawn forwards to bring the laryngeal inlet into view. Once in clear view, a tube can be passed through the rima glottidis and into the trachea.

Accounts of the results of recurrent laryngeal nerve injury in the literature are confusing. Injury to one recurrent laryngeal nerve may result in the affected cord being fixed in either an adducted or abducted position. If the cord is fixed in the adducted position the subject will complain of breathlessness (dyspnoea) on exertion. If the cord is abducted the complaint will be more of hoarseness and weakness of the voice with little or no breathlessness. Bilateral paralysis of the recurrent laryngeal nerves which results in adducted cords causes both dyspnoea and hoarseness.

Damage to the external laryngeal nerve results in paralysis of the cricothyroid muscle. The voice is hoarse since the vocal folds are flabby and 'rubber-band-like'. There is difficulty in singing high notes and the voice tires quickly. Recovery often occurs as the opposite cord and muscle adapt.

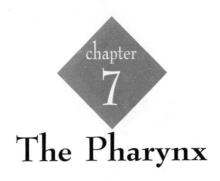

chapter 7

The Pharynx

To see the upper part of the pharynx in its entirety, the ramus of the mandible together with its associated muscles, the parotid salivary gland, and several vessels and cranial nerves must be removed (Fig. 7.1). All of these structures belong to the lower face and will be studied in Section 3.

The pharynx is a muscular tube whose upper muscle fibres arise from the back of the nose on either side, from the **medial pterygoid plates** of the sphenoid bone. It is worth noting now that the lowermost tip of each medial pterygoid plate curves outwards like a hook and is called the **pterygoid hamulus**. The fibres arising on either side from the medial pterygoid plates sweep upwards to the midline posteriorly and attach to the basioccipital bone at a point called the **pharyngeal tubercle**. The muscular tube so formed is part of the **superior constrictor muscle** and this upper part of it bounds the **nasopharynx**.

In the midline posteriorly there is a seam or raphé where the fibres from each side fuse with each other (Fig. 7.2). Muscle fibres of the superior constrictor

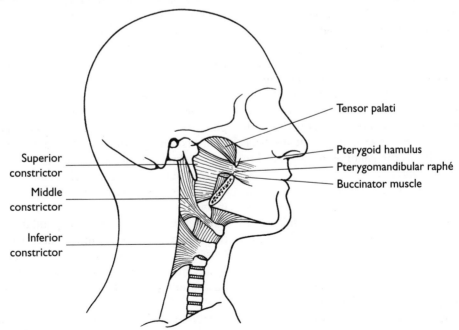

Superior constrictor

Middle constrictor

Inferior constrictor

Tensor palati

Pterygoid hamulus

Pterygomandibular raphé

Buccinator muscle

Figure 7.1 The superior constrictor muscle forms a seam, or raphé, with the buccinator muscle in the cheek. Tensor palati drops from the cranial base outside the superior constrictor and hooks round the pterygoid hamulus into the soft palate.

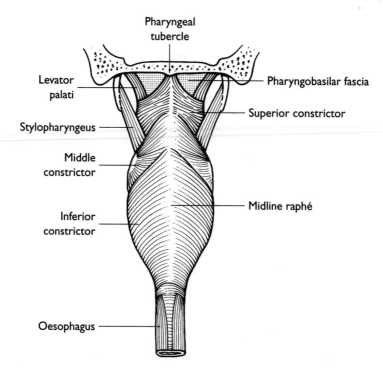

Figure 7.2 The superior, middle and inferior constrictor muscles each run to a midline posterior raphé. The superior constrictor also runs to the bony pharyngeal tubercle. Levator palati pierces the pharyngobasilar fascia to run inside the superior constrictor and into the soft palate. Stylopharyngeus runs between the superior and middle constrictors into the wall of the pharynx.

also arise lower down from the sides of the mouth just below the medial pterygoid plate. They come from another raphé (or line of fusion) extending from the pterygoid hamulus to the inner surface of the mandible on each side of the mouth. This raphé is called the **pterygomandibular raphé** (Fig. 7.1). These muscle fibres of superior constrictor also sweep posteriorly until they fuse together again at the posterior midline raphé of the pharynx. This part of the superior constrictor muscle encircles the **oropharynx** at the back of the oral cavity. It has the **palatine tonsil** applied to its inner wall at the sides.

The **greater horn** of the hyoid bone and the **stylohyoid ligament** give origin to muscle fibres of the **middle constrictor**. These fibres sweep round to the back of the pharynx but run *outside* the lowermost fibres of the superior constrictor muscle at the back to fuse in the midline at the raphé.

Muscle fibres making up the **inferior constrictor muscle** take origin from the sides of the thyroid cartilage and the cricoid cartilage. Once more these fibres sweep backwards, running *outside* the lowermost fibres of the middle constrictor. Posteriorly, they reach the midline raphé. The lowest part of the

pharynx is known as the **laryngopharynx** and lies at the level of the larynx. The midline raphé at the back of the pharynx therefore extends as a continuous seam from the base of the skull at the top to the beginning of the oesophagus below. The three constrictors overlap each other like three stacked flowerpots (Figs 7.1 and 7.2).

Below the inferior constrictor muscle the oesophagus is in continuity with the pharynx. Behind the pharynx and upper part of the oesophagus is the **prevertebral fascia** which covers the prevertebral muscle mass. This is a well-defined layer here and allows free movement of the pharynx and oesophagus independent of prevertebral muscle movement. Between the prevertebral fascia and the posterior wall of the pharynx is a potential space, filled with a little loose connective tissue. It is called the **retropharyngeal space**. Infection in this space can spread rapidly and pus forming here gives rise to a retropharyngeal abscess. You will notice that the framework of the larynx and trachea is cartilaginous whilst that of the pharynx and oesophagus is muscular. Clearly, this reflects the different functional requirements of these two midline tubes. The 'gaps' between the cartilages of the larynx and hyoid are closed by membranes and muscle. You can see from Figure 7.1 that there are also 'gaps' between the pharyngeal muscles at the sides. These are filled with loose connective tissue and, as we shall see, several important structures pass through each gap or space.

Covering the *inner* surfaces of the muscles of the pharynx is the **pharyngobasilar fascia**. This is thin and does not exist in the lower part of the pharynx as a 'membrane', otherwise the pharynx would be unable to expand and contract easily. The outer surface of the pharynx (and cheek) is also covered with a thin layer of epimysium called the **buccopharyngeal membrane**, but this is an insignificant structure beyond facilitating easy movement of the pharynx on the prevertebral fascia. There is a 'gap' between the upper border of the superior constrictor muscle and the cranial base. It is covered over with true membranous pharyngobasilar fascia. Here it extends up from the inside of the pharynx between the free superior edge of the constrictor muscle and the base of the skull (Fig. 7.2).

Two small muscles arise from the base of the skull close to the superior constrictor muscle and proceed to the palate. We will study these in more detail later but notice for the moment their names: **tensor palati** and **levator palati**. The tensor is interesting since it runs down on the outside of the superior constrictor and converges to a delicate tendon which loops around the pterygoid hamulus (Fig. 7.1). It does this in order to change direction and pass horizontally into the palate. The levator palati actually runs over the top of the superior constrictor muscle, through the pharyngobasilar fascia, to reach the top of the palate from the inside of the nasopharynx (Fig. 7.2).

There are other 'gaps' between the upper and middle constrictor muscles of the pharynx and between the middle and inferior constrictor muscles. They are filled with loose connective tissue but also allow important muscles and nerves access to the oropharynx and mouth and to the laryngopharynx and larynx.

The styloid apparatus

Before leaving the external surfaces of the midline tubes we need to study the styloid apparatus (Fig.

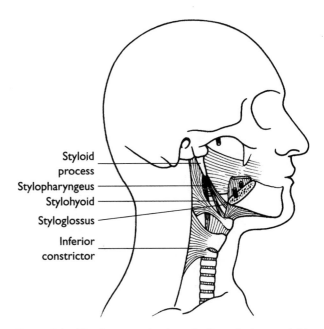

Figure 7.3 The three muscles that arise from the bony styloid process run respectively to the tongue (styloglossus), hyoid bone (stylohyoid) and pharyngeal wall (stylopharyngeus).

7.3). Three muscles arise from the styloid process and pass to the tongue, hyoid bone and pharynx respectively. They are therefore called the **styloglossus**, **stylohyoid** and **stylopharyngeus** muscles.

The styloglossus passes to the tongue between the superior and middle constrictor muscles and acts to pull the tongue upwards and backwards. The stylohyoid emerges more superficially to insert into the hyoid bone at the junction of the body and greater horn. It retracts the hyoid bone in the neck. The stylopharyngeus, however, is a longitudinal muscle of the pharynx. It passes *deep* to the other styloid muscles as it runs from the styloid process and then passes between the internal and external carotids, to enter the wall of the pharynx by passing over the upper border of the middle constrictor (Fig. 7.2). Once inside, it inserts on to the internal surface of the thyroid cartilage. The styloid apparatus concerns us from several points of view. The stylopharyngeus muscle, although delicate, is a guide to the position of the glossopharyngeal nerve (IX). The stylohyoid at its insertion forms an arch through which a tendon belonging to the digastric muscle in the superficial layers of the neck can glide. There is also a stylohyoid ligament which passes deep to this muscle and attaches onto the lesser horn of the hyoid

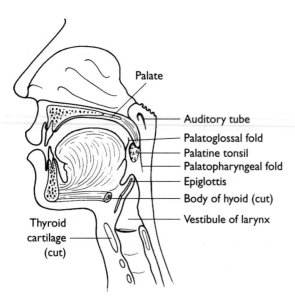

Palate

Auditory tube

Palatoglossal fold

Palatine tonsil

Palatopharyngeal fold

Epiglottis

Body of hyoid (cut)

Vestibule of larynx

Thyroid
cartilage
(cut)

Figure 7.4   The auditory tube opens into the nasopharynx at the level of the floor of the nose. The adenoids lie in the pharyngeal wall behind the soft palate. The palatine tonsil lies between the pillars of the fauces at the entrance to the oropharynx. The laryngopharynx lies behind the epiglottis and vestibule of the larynx.

bone, and we have already seen that this provides some attachment for the middle constrictor muscle at its origin. Finally, the styloglossus is a muscle involved in the delicate and precise movements of the tongue, especially during swallowing and speech.

The interior of the pharynx

The interior of the pharynx is lined with mucous membrane. That in the nasopharynx is respiratory epithelium (pseudostratified ciliated columnar epithelium) whereas the rest of the mucous membrane is stratified squamous epithelium. We have seen previously that the cavity of the pharynx is divided, for descriptive purposes, into three regions. The part behind the nose is the nasopharynx, that posterior to the mouth is the oropharynx and that at the back of the larynx is the laryngopharynx. These relationships can be clearly seen on a paramedian section of the head and neck (Fig. 7.4) or on a lateral skull radiograph of the region. We can now consider these regions in a little more detail.

The nasopharynx lies above the level of the palate. It is continuous below with the oral part through a narrow **pharyngeal isthmus**. In front it communicates with the nasal cavities. The roof and posterior wall consist of mucous membrane covering the bones of the base of the skull. Lymphoid tissue is found in the submucosa of the posterior wall of the pharynx. This is often enlarged in children where aggregations are called '**adenoids**'. If grossly enlarged they can interfere with breathing and often force a child to breathe through an open mouth. This gives the typical appearance called '**adenoidal facies**'.

On the lateral wall of the pharynx at the level of the floor of the nose is the opening of the **auditory tube**. It equalizes the pressure between the pharynx and middle ear and can become blocked in upper respiratory tract infections such as a common cold. The opening for the auditory tube is bounded above and at the back by a **tubal ridge** in which lies more lymphoid tissue. From the ridge, a fold of mucous membrane can be seen descending along the side wall of the pharynx. This fold contains a delicate muscle passing down from the tube to the pharyngeal wall. This is another longitudinal muscle of the pharynx, the **salpingopharyngeus muscle**. Behind the ridge is a deep **pharyngeal recess**.

The oropharynx lies behind the **palatoglossal fold** formed by the **palatoglossus muscle**. Behind this there is another muscle which also raises a fold. This is the **palatopharyngeus muscle**. Sometimes these folds are known as the **anterior** and **posterior pillars of the fauces**. Between the two arches, palatoglossal and palatopharyngeal, lies the **palatine tonsil**. There is one tonsil on either side. They are lymphoid masses and extremely important clinically. The mucous membrane on the surface of the tonsil dips deeply into the substance of the lymphoid tissue to form narrow **tonsillar crypts**. The outer surface of the tonsil is covered by a thin capsule which is attached to the pharyngobasilar fascia and to the sheath of the palatoglossal muscle. This helps to keep the tonsil in place. Outside or lateral to these structures is the superior constrictor muscle. (Note in Figure 5.4 that the facial artery lies outside the superior constrictor muscle here.) The glossopharyngeal nerve is also just lateral to the tonsillar bed. These are all important relations of the tonsil. When the tonsil is removed it has to be cut away from this 'bed'. The blood supply to the tonsil and its venous drainage are important. As would be expected, the chief artery is a branch of the facial artery, which enters the lower part of the tonsil. Veins also pierce the superior constrictor near the artery and either terminate in the pharyngeal plexus of veins or drain into the facial vein. These can bleed badly after tonsillectomy. Lymphatic drainage is through lymphatics which pierce the superior constrictor and go to the nearest lymph nodes. Often these become enlarged and painful in tonsillitis. One node is particularly affected and is called the 'tonsillar' lymph node or **jugulodigastric** lymph node. (We will describe the distribution of lymph nodes in the neck later.)

Two pairs of folds of mucous membrane pass forwards from the epiglottis to the tongue. These are the **median** and two **lateral glossoepiglottic folds**. On either side of the median fold is a depression called the **vallecula**.

The laryngopharynx lies behind the larynx. Its posterior and lateral walls are made up of the middle and inferior constrictors with the lower fibres of the salpingopharyngeus, the palatopharyngeus and stylopharyngeus muscles running longitudinally and internally. Its anterior wall is composed of the inlet of the larynx with the **piriform fossa** or recess on either side. Lower down, the laryngopharynx is made up of the mucous membrane on the back of the cricoid cartilage.

Nerve supply to the pharynx

The neurons that supply the muscles of the pharynx leave the brain through the cranial root of the accessory nerve (XI). These then enter the vagus nerve (X). The various branches of the vagus then distribute the neurons to the muscles. Sensory supply varies with the level of the pharynx. The mucous membrane of the nasopharynx is supplied by the maxillary branch (Vii) of the trigeminal nerve (just like most of the nose). Sensation from the oropharynx is transmitted through the glossopharyngeal nerve (IX) (just like the back of the tongue in fact). The glossopharyngeal nerve also supplies the mucous membrane of the auditory tube. The laryngeal part of the pharynx is supplied by the internal and recurrent branches of the vagus which transmit the sensory neurons back to the brain (just like the larynx). Two of the nerves mentioned above, the pharyngeal branch of the

vagus and the glossopharyngeal nerve (IX), form a plexus with sympathetic fibres on the surface of the pharynx. This is called the **pharyngeal plexus**.

Lymphoid tissue in the pharynx

A glance at the masses of lymphoid tissue around the mouth and pharynx will show that there is a ring of lymphoid tissue surrounding the entrance to the respiratory and digestive tracts (Fig. 7.5). This ring consists of the adenoids (or pharyngeal tonsil) posteriorly behind the soft palate, lymphoid tissue surrounding the opening of the auditory tube, the palatine tonsils on either side and lymphoid tissue at the back of the tongue.

Applied anatomy of the pharynx

An enlarged pharyngeal tonsil can obstruct the auditory tubes and make breathing through the nose difficult. Enlarged palatine tonsils can reduce the size of the oropharyngeal inlet considerably. For these reasons and because the tonsils easily become infected, tonsillectomy is a common operation in children, although less so than previously. A complication of tonsillectomy is bleeding from the tonsillar bed. At least four large arteries contribute to the blood supply of the palatine tonsil and these include the facial, lingual, ascending pharyngeal and palatine arteries (Fig. 7.6). Venous drainage from the palatine tonsil is also copious and postoperative bleeding is often be attributed to a vein from the soft palate (the external palatine vein) that runs through the tonsillar bed. Also deep in the tonsillar bed is the glossopharyngeal nerve as it runs forwards to approach the back of the tongue.

The inferior constrictor muscle and the oesophagus are continuous with one another posterior to the cricoid cartilage. The muscle fibres in this region form what is sometimes called the **cricopharyngeus muscle**. Occasionally, there are inherent weaknesses between the muscles of the pharyngeal wall and oesophagus in this region. In this situation outpouchings from the lumen of the pharynx are then able to protrude through the muscular wall (Fig. 7.7). These **pharyngeal pouches**, or **diverticuli**, are clinically significant because in the first place they collect food and, secondly, a gastroscope may pass into one rather than into the lumen of the oesophagus unless the operator is alert to the chance that a pouch may be present.

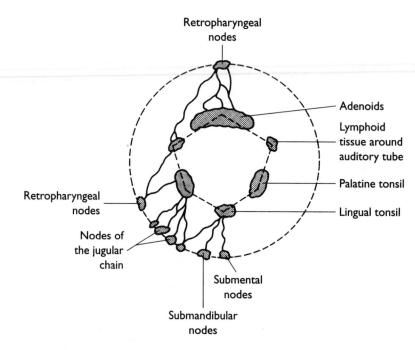

Figure 7.5 Lymphoid tissue surrounds the entrance to the oropharynx. Each mass of lymphoid tissue drains to regional lymph nodes.

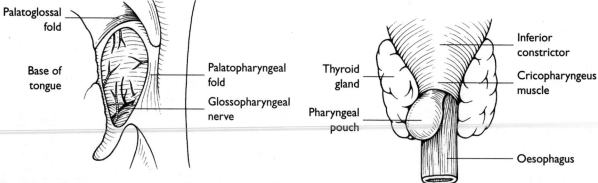

Figure 7.6 The glossopharyngeal nerve lies deep to the tonsillar bed. Tonsillar branches of the lesser palatine, dorsal lingual and ascending pharyngeal vessels each contribute to a rich vascular plexus in the tonsillar bed.

Figure 7.7 Pharyngeal pouches, or diverticula, may herniate through weak regions between the cricopharyngeus muscle fibres and those forming the upper part of the oesophagus.

Superficial Structures of the Neck

The first pair of cervical nerves leaves the spinal cord and vertebral column above the first cervical vertebra, between it and the base of the skull. The remaining seven cervical nerves leave the vertebral column through their corresponding intervertebral foramina. Immediately after leaving an intervertebral foramen each spinal nerve divides into a **dorsal** and **ventral ramus**. The dorsal rami supply the extensor muscles at the back of the neck and the skin overlying them. In the cervical region the upper four ventral rami branch and mix with each other before they pass onwards to skin and muscles. The lower four cervical ventral rami stream towards the upper limb. They join with the first thoracic ventral ramus, and form a plexus which supplies the arm (Fig. 8.1). The upper four ventral rami and their branches form the **cervical plexus**, and the lower four rami together with the first thoracic ramus form the **brachial plexus**.

You will recall that each of the transverse processes of the cervical vertebrae have a foramen in them for the vertebral arteries. Each of these transverse processes also ends in two **tubercles**, an anterior and posterior tubercle. The cervical ventral rami pass out over the transverse processes in a shallow gutter between the anterior and posterior tubercles.

The **scalene muscles**, which run from the cervical vertebral column to the first and second ribs, take origin from these tubercles (Fig. 8.2). The scalene muscles lie at the sides of the vertebral column. The **scalenus anterior** muscle attaches to the anterior tubercles and the **scalenus medius** attaches to the posterior tubercles (along with the **scalenus posterior** and **levator scapulae** in fact). The ventral rami, then,

have to emerge into the neck *between* the scalenus anterior and scalenus medius muscles.

The cervical plexus

The upper four ventral rami give branches that supply many of the muscles in the neck and also the skin of the sides and front of the neck. A few muscular branches from the first cervical ventral ramus enter the hypoglossal nerve and 'hitch-hike' along it. They leave the nerve in the front of the neck as the **superior root of the ansa cervicalis** (Fig. 5.10) and as the **thyrohyoid nerve**. Muscular branches from the second and third ventral rami form the **inferior root of the ansa**. Fine branches from the loop of the ansa pass to the muscles at the front of the neck.

A muscular branch from the fourth ventral ramus needs more careful study. This branch supplies muscle that originally developed in the neck but which later migrated into the thorax. The muscle is, of course, the diaphragm. The branch of the fourth ramus is called the **phrenic nerve**. It receives a few filaments from the third and fifth ventral rami and then passes round on to the surface of the scalenus anterior muscle (Fig. 8.3). From here it crosses it obliquely, passes in front of the subclavian artery and through the superior aperture of the thorax. You will realize, then, that a broken neck above the level of C4 is fatal since the diaphragm will be completely paralysed.

The cutaneous branches from the cervical plexus emerge at the side of the neck and here they radiate

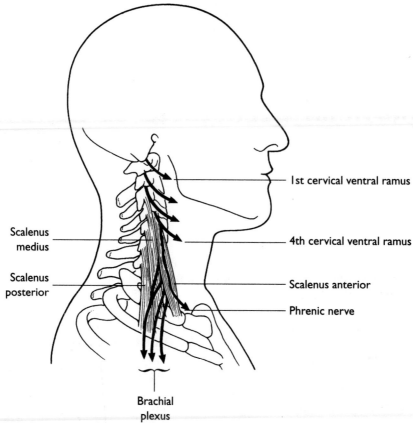

Figure 8.1 The first cervical ventral ramus emerges between the skull and the atlas. Cervical ventral rami forming the cervical and brachial plexuses emerge laterally between the scalenus anterior and scalenus medius muscles.

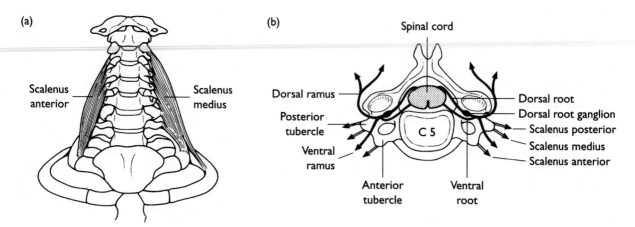

Figure 8.2 The scalene muscles (a) both support the cervical vertebral column and are accessory muscles of respiration. The scalene muscles take origin from the anterior and posterior tubercles of the cervical vertebrae (b).

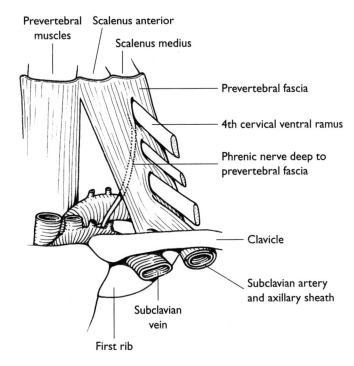

Figure 8.3 The scalene muscles and the prevertebral muscles are covered with prevertebral fascia. The phrenic nerve is located behind this fascia on scalenus anterior. The subclavian artery carries a sheath of this fascia into the axilla (the axillary sheath).

into the skin like the spokes of a wheel (Fig. 8.4). They are named the **lesser occipital, great auricular, transverse cervical** and **supraclavicular nerves**.

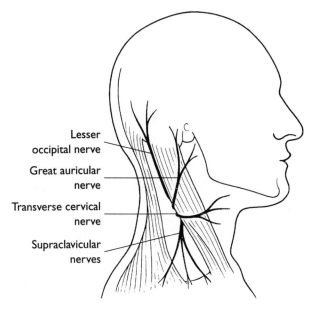

Figure 8.4 The cutaneous nerves of the cervical plexus radiate from the posterior surface of sternocleidomastoid muscle.

The brachial plexus and sympathetic trunk

The fifth, sixth, seventh and eighth ventral rami emerge low in the neck between the scalenus anterior and scalenus medius. Very soon the fifth and sixth rami join together, but the seventh remains separate and then the eighth joins with the first thoracic ramus (Fig. 8.5). Thus three nerve trunks are formed: an **upper**, a **middle** and a **lower trunk**. The three trunks

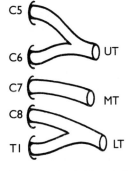

Figure 8.5 The ventral rami of C5 and C6 form the upper trunk of the brachial plexus. C7 forms the middle trunk, and C8 and T1 the lower trunk.

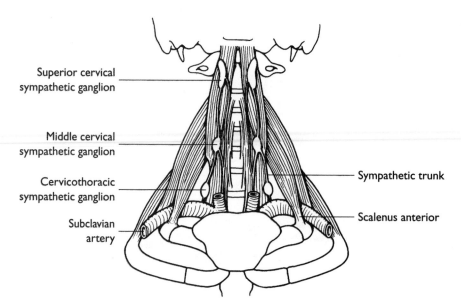

Superior cervical
sympathetic ganglion

Middle cervical
sympathetic ganglion

Cervicothoracic
sympathetic ganglion

Subclavian
artery

Sympathetic trunk

Scalenus anterior

Figure 8.6   There are three cervical sympathetic ganglia in the neck. The cervicothoracic, or stellate, ganglion lies close to the neck of the first rib in the thoracic inlet.

stream over the first rib with the subclavian artery into the upper limb. A sheet of prevertebral fascia covers the prevertebral and scalene muscles. Thus, on emerging from the intervertebral foramina, the cervical ventral rami at first lie deep to this fascia. They therefore have to pierce it in order to reach the structures that they supply. Notice that, in particular, the arrangement in the root of the neck (Fig. 8.3). The brachial plexus and subclavian artery pierce the fascia which bridges the triangular gap between the scalenus anterior and scalenus medius. The artery carries with it a sheath of this fascia into the upper limb, where it is called the **axillary sheath**. The subclavian vein passes over the first rib in front of the scalenus anterior and therefore does not pierce the fascia. One further structure needs to be studied, the cervical part of the sympathetic trunk.

The sympathetic trunk extends from the base of the skull to the superior aperture of the thorax where it is continuous with the thoracic part of the trunk. All the preganglionic neurons in the trunk in this region have *ascended* from the thoracic region. Remember that there is no preganglionic outflow from the cervical part of the cord. The neurons ascend to one of three cervical sympathetic ganglia on the trunk. They are named the **superior**, **middle** and **inferior cervical sympathetic ganglia**. Often the inferior ganglion is fused with the first thoracic ganglion to form a large **cervicothoracic ganglion** (sometimes called the **stellate ganglion**

because of its flattened star-like appearance). This lies on the neck of the first rib (Fig. 8.6).

Postganglionic sympathetic fibres arise in all three ganglia and many of them climb along blood vessels to reach their destination in the head and neck. Fibres from the superior ganglion climb the internal and external carotids. Fibres from the middle ganglion climb along the inferior thyroid arteries and those from the lower ganglion climb along the vertebral artery. A few postganglionic fibres descend from each ganglion on the prevertebral fascia back into the thorax as **cardiac branches**. These are destined to go through the cardiac plexus and to the heart. Some postganglionic fibres pass from ganglia back into the cervical ventral rami and then are distributed with them to the skin of the neck and upper limb. A slender branch from the middle ganglion loops around the subclavian artery and rejoins the cervicothoracic ganglion. It is called the **ansa subclavia** and gives some sympathetic fibres to the subclavian artery destined for the upper limb.

Only one structure needs to be added on the left side to complete the picture of the root of the neck. This is the **thoracic duct**. This duct ascends from the thorax behind the oesophagus on top of the prevertebral fascia. Here, in the root of the neck, it arches forwards to enter the venous system at the junction of the left internal jugular and left subclavian veins (Fig. 8.7).

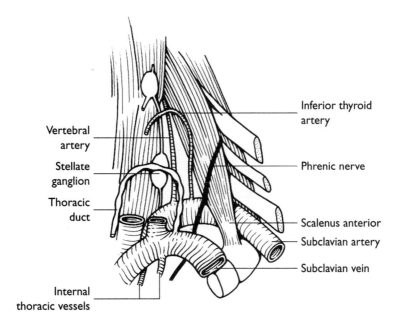

Vertebral artery

Stellate ganglion

Thoracic duct

Internal thoracic vessels

Inferior thyroid artery

Phrenic nerve

Scalenus anterior

Subclavian artery

Subclavian vein

Figure 8.7 Scalenus anterior attaches to the first rib between the subclavian vein and subclavian artery. The thoracic duct arches over and drains into the junction between the internal jugular vein and the subclavian vein here in the root of the neck.

Musculofascial coverings in the neck

A thin sheet of muscle is found in the subcutaneous fat of the neck. It is called the **platysma muscle**. Platysma is really a muscle of facial expression supplied by the facial nerve (VII). Its fibres arise from the deep fascia and skin on the front of the chest and shoulder, and sweep upwards over the front and sides of the neck. They insert into the deep fascia of the neck, the lower border of the mandible and the deep fascia of the lower face.

Deep to the subcutaneous fat and the platysma there are two large muscles enclosed within the investing fascia of the neck. These muscles are the **sternocleidomastoid** and **trapezius** (Fig. 8.8). The sternocleidomastoid arises from the front of the manubrium by a round tendon and from the medial third of the clavicle as a flat muscular sheet. The two sets of fibres fuse on their way upwards to the mastoid process of the skull and the lateral part of the superior nuchal line on the back of the occipital bone. The deep surface of the sternocleidomastoid muscle is pierced by the spinal part of the accessory nerve (XI) which supplies motor neurons to the muscle.

Acting alone, one sternocleidomastoid will flex the cervical column laterally and draw the head down to that side. At the same time, however, it also rotates the head on the cervical column so that the face is turned up towards the opposite side. When both muscles act together they flex the cervical column and head forwards.

Only the anterior edge of the trapezius can be seen from the front. The muscle is best seen from the side and back (Fig. 8.8). The trapezius arises from the middle of the superior nuchal line and from the spines of the cervical and thoracic vertebrae. Its fibres sweep towards the shoulder where they are inserted into the lateral third of the clavicle, the acromion process of the scapula and the spine of the scapula. The muscle is also supplied by the accessory nerve (XI) and its action is on the shoulder. It can be tested by asking the subject to shrug their shoulders. The detailed actions of trapezius are usually studied in detail with the upper limb.

The two muscles just described leave two triangular-shaped 'windows' in the investing layer of fascia. They are called the **anterior** and **posterior triangles** of the neck. The anterior triangle has its base at the top in the form of the lower border of the mandible. The posterior triangle has its base below in the form of the middle third of the clavicle. In fact, the two triangular gaps are covered over with deep

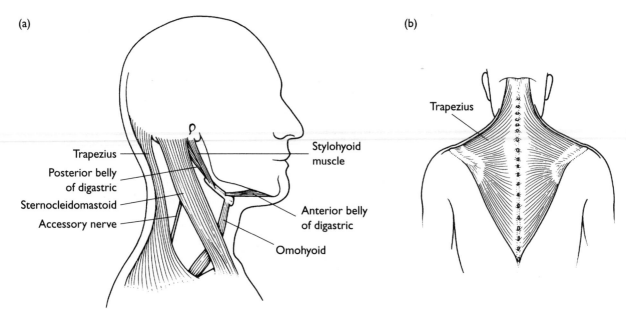

Figure 8.8   The posterior triangle is bounded by the anterior border of trapezius and the posterior border of the sternocleidomastoid. The anterior triangle lies anterior to the anterior borders of the sternocleidomastoid muscles in the anterior midline of the neck.

investing cervical fascia (look back to Figure 5.1 to see this).

By far the most important structure in the posterior triangle of the neck is the accessory nerve, the XIth cranial nerve. This nerve enters the deep aspect of the sternocleidomastoid muscle close to the mastoid process. It then leaves the substance of the sternocleidomastoid muscle about one-third of the way down its posterior border. The accessory nerve travels obliquely downwards and backwards across the posterior triangle to enter the trapezius muscle about one-third of the way up its anterior border (Fig. 8.8). As it crosses the posterior triangle the accessory nerve lies within the deep investing fascia of the neck.

This so-called deep fascia is complete around the neck. It invests the neck from mandible above to clavicle below. The fascia actually encloses the sternocleidomastoid and trapezius muscles, and extends around the back of the neck to cover the extensor muscles in that region as well. In the midline below, it splits into two layers that are attached to the front and back of the manubrium. There is thus a 'suprasternal space' in this region containing a little fatty tissue and a vein passing through it from side to side.

The strap muscles

When the investing deep fascia and the sternocleidomastiod muscles are removed, several small strap-like muscles are revealed underneath. Three of these lie to the side of the midline in the front of the neck and two run across the sides of the neck (Fig. 8.9). The strap muscles lie on either side of the midline below the hyoid and in front of the laryngeal cartilages and thyroid gland. The **sternohyoid muscle** can clearly be seen passing from the back of the manubrium below to the hyoid bone above (Fig. 8.9). If the two muscles are removed, a deeper set of strap muscles is brought into view. These are the **sternothyroid** and **thyrohyoid muscles**. The sternothyroid passes from the back of the manubrium to the oblique line on the thyroid cartilage and the thyrohyoid from this oblique line onwards to the lower border of the hyoid.

The nerve supply to the strap muscles is from the upper cervical ventral rami. These are the fibres of C1 that 'hitch-hiked' along the hypoglossal nerve. They leave the nerve as the superior root of the ansa cervicalis. The other rami give fibres as the inferior root of the ansa and these two roots join as a 'U' shaped loop on the common carotid artery and internal jugular vein. Branches from the ansa enter

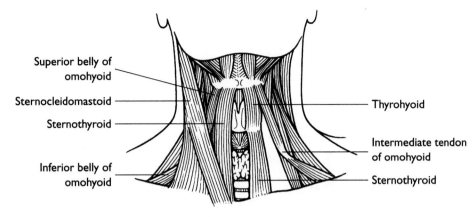

Figure 8.9 When the sternocleidomastoid muscle is removed, the strap muscles at the front of the neck are revealed overlying the thyroid cartilage and thyroid gland.

the strap muscles. A small nerve containing only C1 fibres leaves the hypoglossal nerve separately and enters the **thyrohyoid muscle** and the **geniohyoid muscle** independent of the ansa (Fig. 5.10).

The strap muscles act on the hyoid bone and larynx. They can depress the hyoid or, with the aid of the muscles in the floor of the mouth, they can fix the hyoid. Fixation produces a stable bony basis on which the tongue can move. Their action on the larynx is seen during swallowing. The thyrohyoid first elevates the thyroid cartilage towards the hyoid, then the sternothyroid depresses the larynx. This rise and fall of the larynx can clearly be seen in the neck during each swallow.

Two other muscles in the neck each have two bellies. These are the **digastric** and the **omohyoid muscles** (Figs 8.8 and 8.9). The bellies of each of these muscles are united by a small **intermediate tendon**. The tendon, in both cases, slides through a small fibrous fascial sling. In the case of the digastric muscle, the anterior belly arises from a depression on the mandible beneath the chin. The posterior belly arises from a notch on the medial side of the mastoid process on the cranial base. The fibrous pulley through which the intermediate tendon runs is attached to the hyoid bone. The tendon is surrounded by a synovial sheath to minimize friction.

The two bellies of the digastric muscle are supplied by two different nerves, an indication of their differing developmental origins. The anterior belly derives its nerve supply from a small branch of the mandibular division of the trigeminal nerve (Viii). This nerve supplies the **mylohyoid muscle** in the floor of the mouth as well as the anterior belly of digastric.

The posterior belly is supplied by the facial nerve (VII).

The action of the digastric muscle depends on whether or not the hyoid bone is fixed. Acting on an unfixed hyoid, the muscle raises that bone, an action seen during swallowing. On the other hand, acting with the infrahyoid strap muscles on a fixed hyoid bone, it opens the mouth by lowering the mandible.

The omohyoid muscle has superior and inferior bellies which are also united by an intermediate tendon. The inferior belly arises from the upper part of the scapula and passes forwards over the root of the neck. Its superior belly arises from the inferior border of the hyoid bone. The intermediate tendon passes through a fascial sling which is attached to the fascia on the deep surface of the sternocleidomastoid muscle (Fig. 8.9). The muscle acts on the hyoid bone in exactly the same way as the strap muscles. It also has the same nerve supply as these muscles.

Lymph nodes in the neck

Many lymph nodes in the neck lie in close relationship to the jugular vein and to either the digastric or omohyoid muscles. Those lying above the digastric belong to the floor of the mouth and will be studied with the structures in this section. A deep group of cervical lymph nodes is strung along the internal jugular vein and carotid sheath. This group receives lymph from other more superficial groups of regional lymph nodes in the neck. The regional groups of

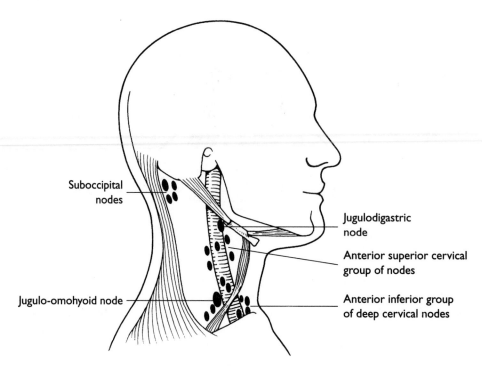

Suboccipital
nodes

Jugulodigastric
node

Anterior superior cervical
group of nodes

Jugulo-omohyoid node

Anterior inferior group
of deep cervical nodes

Figure 8.10 A deep chain of lymph nodes lies along the internal jugular vein and carotid sheath. More superficial regional nodes are found posterior to this and anterior to this chain, but eventually all drain into them.

lymph nodes of the neck are divided descriptively into four groups (Fig. 8.10). The nodes lying behind the internal jugular vein are the **posterior nodes** and those in front are the **anterior nodes**. The upper members of each group are called the **superior nodes** and the lower members the **inferior nodes**. One node that lies in the angle between the digastric and jugular vein is called the **jugulodigastric node**. We saw that the tonsil and the back of the tongue drain lymph into this node, which often becomes painful and enlarged during tonsillitis. It is one of the ante-rosuperior group. The anteroinferior group lie just above the clavicle and are usually called the **supra-clavicular nodes**. They are important since some of the trunk and upper limb lymph drains through them on its way to the great neck veins. Thus cancer of the breast which has a secondary deposit in a supraclavicular node has already invaded the thoracic cavity through the internal thoracic nodes. Sometimes a secondary deposit is found in a supraclavicular node from carcinoma of the stomach. Another named node of the posteroinferior group is the jugulo-omohyoid node.

Cutaneous nerves and superficial veins in the neck

Venous drainage from the lower facial region and the temple passes downwards into the neck through the **retromandibular vein** and the **posterior auricular vein** (Fig. 8.11). Deep to the parotid gland the retro-mandibular vein divides into anterior and posterior branches. The posterior branch joins the posterior auricular vein to form the **external jugular vein**. The external jugular vein proceeds down through the sub-cutaneous tissue of the neck on the surface of the sternocleidomastoid muscle. It pierces the investing layer of deep cervical fascia towards the base of the posterior triangle and travels deeply to empty into the **internal jugular vein**. The anterior branch of the retromandibular vein joins the **facial vein** which pierces the cervical fascia to enter the internal jugular vein. Draining the superficial tissues of the floor of the mouth and the front of the neck are two veins called the **anterior jugular veins** (Fig. 8.12). The anterior jugular veins drain down and pierce the fascia of the anterior triangle just above the manubrium. Here they enter the suprasternal fascial

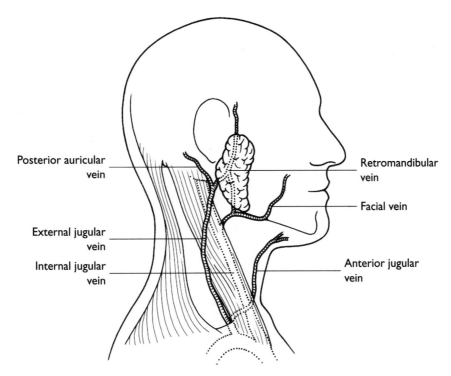

Figure 8.11 The most common superficial venous drainage pattern of the face and side of the neck.

space. In this space the two veins are joined across the midline by a **jugular venous arch**. The suprasternal space and jugular arch are encountered during exposure of the thyroid gland or upper trachea during surgery. The arch is often quite large. The anterior jugular veins themselves continue laterally, deep to the sternocleidomastoid to join the external jugular veins which have already pierced the deep fascia.

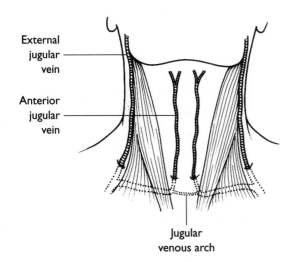

Figure 8.12 The most common pattern of superficial venous drainage in the front of the neck.

We have already described the cutaneous branches of the cervical ventral rami (Fig. 8.4). They appear subcutaneously along the posterior border of the sternocleidomastoid muscle. They radiate like the spokes of a wheel into the tissues of the neck. The lesser occipital nerve passes up to skin over the back of the ear and to skin of the scalp behind the ear. The great auricular nerve spreads out into skin over the front and back of the ear. The transverse cervical nerve supplies skin on the front and side of the neck. The supraclavicular nerves pass down over the clavicle as medial, intermediate and lateral nerves to supply the front of the chest. They can be palpated in the living as they pass over the bony clavicle.

Applied anatomy of the neck

It is a good anatomical exercise to consider the possible origin of lumps in the neck (Fig. 8.13). Midline swellings in the neck can be associated with the thyroid gland and often reflect its development. An enlarged thyroid gland, or **goitre,** is able to expand down through the thoracic inlet but unable to rise any higher in the neck than the oblique line of the thyroid cartilage. This is because the attachment of

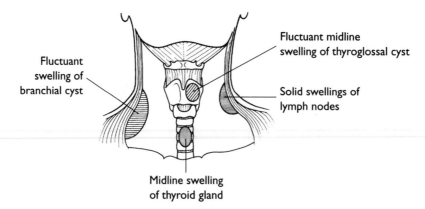

Fluctuant swelling of branchial cyst

Fluctuant midline swelling of thyroglossal cyst

Solid swellings of lymph nodes

Midline swelling of thyroid gland

Figure 8.13 Swellings in the neck may be fluctuant or soild, fixed or mobile. Swellings of thyroid origin are common midline swellings, and rise and fall on swallowing. Lymph nodes more laterally may be indicative of infection or neoplasm. Rarely, congenital swellings present in the neck.

the thyrohyoid muscle prevents the gland expanding upwards. Since the thyroid is tied to the trachea by pretracheal fascia it moves up and down in the neck during swallowing.

Thyroglossal cysts can occur anywhere along the developmental path of migration of the thyroid gland and are another common cause of fluctuant midline swellings in the neck. Lymph nodes are often enlarged in the neck. They may be due to anything from tonsillitis to tuberculosis or even carcinoma. The chains of lymph nodes in the neck lie along the internal jugular vein and can be felt at the anterior border of the sternocleidomastoid muscle. A ring of smaller lymph nodes lies around the neck like a collar from the occipital region to the submandibular region and to the submental region.

Branchial cysts result during development when the rapidly growing second arch overlaps the lower pharyngeal arches but then the ectoderm of the second arch fails to fuse higher up and fuses only with the lowermost arches (Fig. 8.14). This leaves a cervical sinus with ectodermal walls which then slowly fill with fluid and eventually present as a discrete swelling in the neck during childhood. Branchial cysts protrude from the anterior border of the sternocleidomastoid muscle just below the angle of the mandible.

Tracheostomy is an elective procedure performed to reduce the dead space in the airway of a weak patient or to facilitate prolonged artificial ventilation of patients. This procedure illustrates the anatomy of the neck in the midline in a practical way (Fig. 8.15). A transverse incision is made in the neck through

skin and platysma (that is in same direction as the skin creases) midway between the cricoid cartilage and the suprasternal notch. The strap muscles are then retracted to each side and the isthmus of the thyroid gland identified. This is extremely vascular and is clamped, ligatured and divided. The trachea beneath is opened below the first tracheal ring and a flap raised and hinged over inferiorly. Its free edge is then sewn to the skin to ensure clear access to the airway.

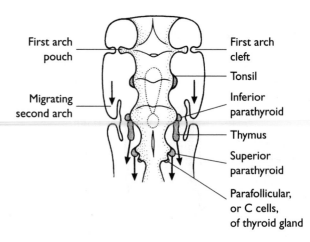

First arch pouch

Migrating second arch

First arch cleft

Tonsil

Inferior parathyroid

Thymus

Superior parathyroid

Parafollicular, or C cells, of thyroid gland

Figure 8.14 Branchial cysts arise during development when the rapidly growing second arch overlaps the lower pharyngeal arches, but then the ectoderm of the second arch fails to fuse with that underlying it higher up, fusing only with the lowermost arches. This encloses a potential space that may become filled with fluid. The derivatives of the pharyngeal pouches are also indicated in the figure.

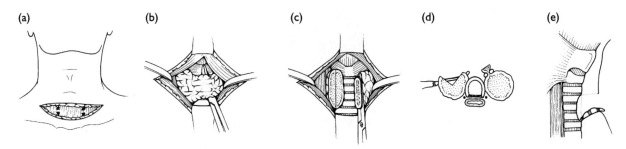

Figure 8.15 Stages of an elective tracheostomy. See text for description. (After Hollinshead WH (1982) *Anatomy for Surgeons.* Philadelphia: Harper and Row.)

chapter 9

Summary and Revision of the Pharynx, Larynx and Neck

First read through the following summaries of the cranial nerves that run down through the neck and that we have studied in the last three chapters. Be sure you are clear about their course, what they supply and how they can be tested. Use Figure 9.1 to help you recall each one. Some of the multiple choice questions that follow require a knowledge of facts given in these summaries. Next, to bring together what you have learned about the neck, the larynx and the pharynx, go through the multiple choice questions at the end of this chapter. For each **stem**, any one of the five answers (A)–(E) may be either correct or incorrect. You may choose to do them all on one occasion or you may choose to do alternate questions at your first attempt. Many of these questions are intentionally quite searching. A score of around 50% correct would be quite reasonable at your first attempt. We expect you to have to refer back to the text to improve your score on subsequent attempts. In so doing you will improve your understanding of head and neck anatomy.

Summary of cranial nerves IX, X, XI and XII

Cranial nerve IX

The glossopharyngeal nerve leaves the skull through the jugular foramen in the posterior cranial fossa. The nerve has two sensory ganglia which contain the cell bodies of the sensory nerve fibres. One of these lies in the jugular foramen and the other just below it. The glossopharyngeal nerve passes down the neck between the internal and external carotid arteries. It travels here with the stylopharyngeus, which it supplies. It then passes

between the superior and middle constrictor muscles to enter the side of the pharynx deep to the palatine tonsillar bed. From here it runs to the back of the tongue. A branch from the region of the inferior sensory ganglion passes up into the middle ear cavity and then reforms on the medial wall of the cavity as the lesser superficial petrosal nerve. This runs out through the front of the petrous temporal bone and then down and out of the skull again through the foramen ovale. The glossopharyngeal nerve supplies the baroreceptors in the region of the carotid sinus and the chemoreceptors in the carotid body. Pharyngeal branches contribute sensory nerve fibres to the pharyngeal plexus. The glossopharyngeal nerve is sensory to the back of the oropharynx. The nerve may be tested by stimulating the back of the oropharynx. The 'gag reflex' that results is assurance that the sensory nerve supply to this region is intact.

Cranial nerve X

The vagus nerve passes out of the skull through the jugular foramen. It also has two ganglia here that contain the cell bodies of the sensory nerve fibres of the vagus. The vagus passes down the neck in the carotid sheath, first with the internal carotid artery and then with the common carotid artery. Its first branch is the auricular branch that runs up again through the petrous temporal bone to supply the skin behind the ear and the posterior wall of the external auditory meatus. (Irritating this nerve in, for example, operations that involve the ear may cause vomiting through a vagal reflex.) Pharyngeal branches of the vagus contribute motor nerve fibres to the pharyngeal plexus and also supply the levator palati muscle. The superior laryngeal nerve arises high in the neck and travels down behind the internal carotid artery. It then divides into the external laryngeal nerve, which is motor to the criocothyroid muscle, and the internal laryngeal nerve, which is sensory to the mucosa of the larynx above the level of the vocal folds. The main vagal trunk passes into the thoracic inlet and can be found in the thorax lying against the trachea on the right and on the aortic arch on the

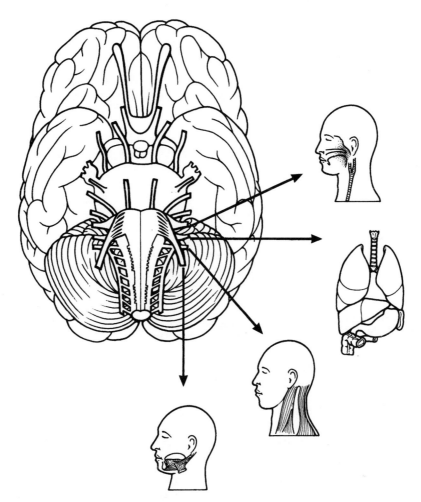

Figure 9.1 Summary of the cranial nerves studied in chapters 5, 6, 7 and 8.

left. The recurrent laryngeal nerves recur, respectively, around the aorta on the left and the subclavian artery on the right. They supply all intrinsic muscles of the larynx except cricothyroid and sensation to the mucous membrane of the larynx below the level of the vocal folds. The vagus nerve in the neck can be tested by asking a subject to raise their soft palate (say ahh!) and to swallow, and by checking that the sensory nerve supply to the piriform fossa and epiglottis is intact.

Cranial nerve XI

The accessory nerve arises both from the upper cervical spinal segments (the spinal accessory) and from the medulla (cranial accessory). The spinal accessory passes up through the foramen magnum and into the posterior cranial fossa. Both parts of the nerve then leave the posterior fossa through the jugular foramen in company with the vagus and glossopharyngeal nerve. The fibres of the cranial accessory immediately join the vagus nerve and are distributed to the pharyngeal plexus and through the larngeal nerves with it. The spinal accessory nerve quickly runs into the deep surface of sternocleidomastoid muscle, which it

supplies with motor fibres, and then runs out of this muscle across the posterior triangle of the neck and into trapezius, which it also supplies. The spinal accessory muscle can be tested by asking a subject to shrug their shoulders against resistance from your hands, and to turn their face against the palm of your hand. The force of each of the muscles can be judged in this way. The right sternocleidomastoid muscle turns the face to the left and vice versa.

Cranial nerve XII

The hypoglossal nerve leaves the skull through the foramen magnum but then immediately enters the hypoglossal canal just above the occipital condyle. The nerve swings outwards and laterally behind the vagus and both the internal and external carotid arteries. At the level of the hyoid bone the hypoglossal nerve runs forwards and joins the lingual artery. Its course in the floor of the mouth will be described later. The nerve is the motor nerve to all of the muscles of the tongue except palatoglossus. It can be tested by asking a subject to stick their tongue out. The tongue deviates to the side of any lesion of the hypoglossal nerve.

Multiple Choice Questions on the Neck, Larynx and Pharynx

1. Structures passing through the jugular foramen include:
(A) the hypoglossal nerve
(B) the vagus nerve
(C) the straight sinus
(D) the glossopharyngeal nerve
(E) the vertebral artery

A____ B____ C____ D____ E____

2. Structures passing through the foramen magnum include:
(A) the basilar artery
(B) the spinal accessory nerves
(C) the dura mater
(D) the hypoglossal nerves (XII)
(E) the internal vertebral venous plexus

A____ B____ C____ D____ E____

3. The scalenus anterior muscle:
(A) is attached to the scalene tubercle of the first rib
(B) is active during deep inspiration
(C) lies anterior to the subclavian vein
(D) has the vagus nerve on its anterior surface
(E) lies anterior to the nerves forming the brachial plexus

A____ B____ C____ D____ E____

4. The subclavian artery:
(A) grooves the bone of the first rib in front of scalenus anterior
(B) is a branch of the common carotid artery on the right
(C) has the recurrent laryngeal nerve beneath it on the right
(D) gives off both superior and inferior thyroid arteries
(E) gives rise to the vertebral artery

A____ B____ C____ D____ E____

5. The phrenic nerve:
(A) gives motor fibres to the diaphragm
(B) contains sensory fibres
(C) arises from ventral rami of cervical spinal nerves
(D) contains some nerve fibres whose cell bodies are in the spinal ganglion of C4 spinal nerve
(E) leaves the neck in the axillary sheath

A____ B____ C____ D____ E____

6. The vagus nerve in the neck:
(A) transmits sympathetic fibres
(B) passes through the foramen magnum
(C) innervates the mucous membrane of the larynx
(D) innervates tongue muscles
(E) innervates pharyngeal muscles

A____ B____ C____ D____ E____

7. The external carotid artery:
(A) is a branch of the internal carotid artery
(B) divides into the superficial temporal and maxillary arteries
(C) supplies the retina via the ophthalmic artery
(D) gives a branch to the thyroid gland
(E) supplies a branch to the tongue

A____ B____ C____ D____ E____

8. Concerning the carotid body and the carotid sinus:
(A) the carotid sinus lies opposite the cricoid cartilage
(B) the carotid sinus is sensitive to changes in arterial blood pressure
(C) the carotid sinus is innervated by the vagus nerve
(D) the carotid body lies beneath the endothelium, within the posterior wall of the common carotid artery
(E) the carotid body is innervated by the vagus nerve

A____ B____ C____ D____ E____

9. The thyroid gland:
(A) has an isthmus lying over the cricoid cartilage
(B) receives a blood supply from branches of the internal carotid artery
(C) lies deep to the sternothyroid muscles
(D) may have a blood supply from a branch of the aorta
(E) rises and falls in the neck during swallowing

A____ B____ C____ D____ E____

10. The thyroid gland:
(A) develops as a midline structure in the floor of embryological pharynx
(B) occasionally has a small pyramidal lobe in the midline superiorly
(C) is completely enclosed in pretracheal fascia
(D) completely encircles the trachea
(E) has veins which drain into the left brachiocephalic vein

A____ B____ C____ D____ E____

11. The right recurrent laryngeal nerve:
(A) is closely related to the right inferior thyroid artery
(B) supplies the posterior cricoarytenoid muscle
(C) supplies the right cricothyroid muscle
(D) carries sensation from the mucous membrane of the piriform fossa
(E) carries sensation from mucous membrane on the back of the epiglottis

A____ B____ C____ D____ E____

12. In the larynx:
(A) the posterior cricoarytenoid muscle is supplied by the external laryngeal nerve
(B) the cricoid cartilage is a complete ring of cartilage
(C) the vocal ligaments are tensed by contraction of the cricothyroid muscle
(D) sensation below the level of the vocal folds is supplied by the recurrent laryngeal nerve
(E) the cricothyroid ligament lies above the level of the vocal folds

A____ B____ C____ D____ E____

13. The vocal fold:
(A) lies beneath the level of the vestibular fold
(B) is covered by ciliated columnar epithelium
(C) is tensed by the aryepiglottic muscle
(D) is relaxed by the cricothyroid muscle
(E) is found at the level of the cricoid cartilage

A____ B____ C____ D____ E____

14. Muscles capable of elevating the larynx are:
(A) omohyoid
(B) digastric
(C) sternothyroid
(D) stylohyoid
(E) stylopharyngeus

A____ B____ C____ D____ E____

15. The superior constrictor of the pharynx:
(A) has fibres that originate from the lateral pterygoid plate
(B) has fibres that originate from the pterygomandibular raphé
(C) inserts above into the pharyngeal tubercle on the occipital bone
(D) has fibres that lie outside those of the middle constrictor
(E) is supplied with motor fibres from the glossopharyngeal nerve

A____ B____ C____ D____ E____

16. The palatine tonsil:
(A) is covered by stratified squamous epithelium
(B) has a lymphatic drainage to the jugulodigastric lymph node
(C) receives its main blood supply from the maxillary artery
(D) lies in a fossa bounded by the palatoglossus and the palatopharyngeous muscles
(E) lies on a 'bed' formed by the middle constrictor of the pharynx

A____ B____ C____ D____ E____

17. The internal jugular vein:
(A) has valves
(B) descends through the neck in the carotid sheath
(C) receives blood from the thyroid gland
(D) has a chain of lymph nodes lying along its course
(E) is crossed by the accessory nerve

A____ B____ C____ D____ E____

18. The ansa cervicalis:
(A) runs around the subclavian artery on the right
(B) gives branches that innervate the omohyoid muscle
(C) gives branches that innervate the sternohyoid muscle
(D) gives sensory branches to the skin over the larynx
(E) contains nerve fibres whose segmental origin is C1, C2 and C3

A____ B____ C____ D____ E____

19 The stylomastoid foramen:
(A) transmits the middle meningeal artery
(B) lies in the occipital bone
(C) opens into the middle ear cavity
(D) transmits the facial nerve
(E) transmits the vestibulocochlear (VIIIth cranial) nerve

A____ B____ C____ D____ E____

20. The posterior triangle of the neck:
(A) is bounded posteriorly by the anterior border of trapezius
(B) is bounded anteriorly by the scalenus anterior muscle
(C) has the spinal part of the accessory nerve (XI) running across it
(D) contains the roots of the brachial plexus as they pass between scalenus anterior and scalenus medius
(E) is bounded inferiorly by the first rib

A____ B____ C____ D____ E____

21. The facial nerve:
(A) supplies the posterior belly of the digastric muscle
(B) contains taste fibres from the posterior third of the tongue
(C) is deep to the retromandibular vein in the parotid gland
(D) leaves the skull through the stylomastoid foramen
(E) contains parasympathetic nerve fibres that innervate the dilator pupillae

A____ B____ C____ D____ E____

22. The external carotid artery:
(A) is crossed superficially by the hypoglossal nerve
(B) usually divides into its terminal branches at the level of the hyoid bone
(C) makes a considerable contribution to the cerebral circulation
(D) is the only source of blood to the thyroid gland
(E) supplies blood to muscles of facial expression

A____ B____ C____ D____ E____

23. The following structures lie between the external and internal carotid arteries:

(A) the glossopharyngeal nerve
(B) the superior laryngeal nerve
(C) the stylohyoid muscle
(D) the pharyngeal branch of the vagus nerve
(E) the styloglossus muscle

A____ B____ C____ D____ E____

24. The glossopharyngeal nerve:

(A) is entirely sensory
(B) leaves the skull through the jugular foramen
(C) supplies a branch to the tympanic plexus
(D) is closely related to the stylopharyngeus muscle in the neck
(E) supplies mucous membrane of the oropharynx

A____ B____ C____ D____ E____

25. Nerves of the cervical plexus:

(A) arise from cervical segments C1 to C8
(B) emerge between scalenus anterior and scalenus medius
(C) include the phrenic nerve
(D) are sensory to the skin overlying the clavicles
(E) include the spinal accessory nerve

A____ B____ C____ D____ E____

Answers to Multiple Choice Questions

1. A F B T C F D T E F	10. A T B T C T D F E T	19. A F B F C F D T E F
2. A F B T C T D T E T	11. A T B T C F D F E F	20. A T B F C T D T E F
3. A T B T C F D F E T	12. A F B T C T D T E F	21. A T B F C F D T E F
4. A F B F C T D F E T	13. A F B F C F D F E F	22. A T B F C F D F E T
5. A T B T C T D T E F	14. A F B T C F D T E T	23. A T B F C F D T E F
6. A F B F C T D F E T	15. A F B T C T D F E F	24. A F B T C T D T E T
7. A F B T C F D T E T	16. A T B T C F D T E F	25. A F B T C T D T E F
8. A F B T C F D F E F	17. A T B T C T D T E T	
9. A F B F C T D T E T	18. A F B T C T D T E T	

THE NOSE, MOUTH AND FACE

The Nose and Paranasal Air Sinuses

First we need to study the bones that form the framework of the nose and face since this is the key to a good understanding of the region (Figs 10.1 and 10.2). The **maxilla** occupies a large region of the skull in the angle between the orbit and nose, and thus forms a great part of the framework of the face. In spite of its size it is a fairly frail bone because its inside is excavated by a large air sinus. This is the **maxillary air sinus** or **antrum**. Notice how the maxilla forms most of the floor of the orbit and the

lateral wall of the nose. A bony tunnel runs through the floor of the orbit. This is called the **infraorbital canal** which opens on to the face at the **infraorbital foramen**.

Two bones that articulate with the maxilla need careful examination. These are the **zygomatic bone** and the **sphenoid bone**. The zygomatic bone is easily palpable on the living face. It forms most of the 'cheek bone'. It takes part in the formation of the lateral wall of the bony orbit and also of the zygomatic arch. The

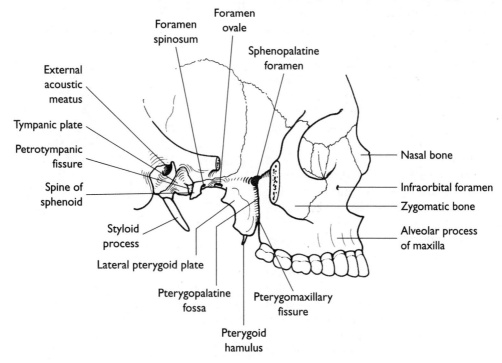

Figure 10.1   The bones and bony landmarks of the face and infratemporal fossa.

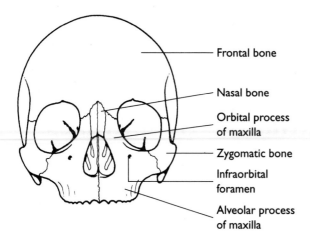

Figure 10.2 The bones of the face seen from the front.

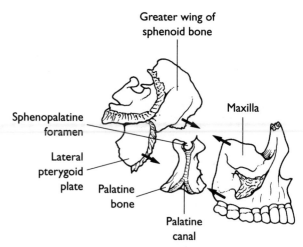

Figure 10.3 The palatine bone is wedged between the sphenoid bone and the maxilla. The vertical part of the palatine bone is forked superiorly and forms the lower part of the sphenopalatine foramen. The palatine canal runs down against the palatine bone towards the hard palate.

greater and lesser wings of the sphenoid bone are visible at the back of the orbital cavity. The greater wing extends laterally to contribute to the side of the cranium. The undersurface of the sphenoid is irregular and extends down to the level of the sides of the soft palate in the form of two plates called the **lateral** and **medial pterygoid plates.**

Between the sphenoid and the maxilla there is a slit where the bones do not quite meet. This is called the **pterygomaxillary fissure.** Deeper within this fissure is another bone that lies opposite the pterygoid plates of the sphenoid bone. This is a part of the **palatine bone** (Fig. 10.3). For this reason the deepest part of the fissure is renamed the **pterygopalatine fossa.** Look for this on a skull and understand that it has several bony tunnels leading into its deepest part. From inside the skull there are two entrances into the fossa, one large and one smaller, but both lead out of the middle cranial fossa.

Identify the **foramen rotundum**, a round hole in the sphenoid bone (Figs 10.4 and 10.5). The foramen rotundum lies below the superior orbital fissure. The opening of the smaller **pterygoid canal** is below this level. It is hidden from view in an articulated skull. Like the foramen rotundum the pterygoid canal passes right through the sphenoid bone from its posterior surface and opens into the pterygopalatine fossa anteriorly. Identify these two foramina on a disarticulated sphenoid bone if you can. It is also useful to pass a fine thread or wire into each and confirm for yourself that they enter the pterygopalatine fossa. Look at Figure 10.5, where the sphenoid bone has been removed from the middle cranial fossa of the skull, and you are looking at it from behind. Again,

note the pterygoid canal and the foramen rotundum, which both lead to the pterygopalatine fossa. The infraorbital fissure and canal continue onwards to the infraorbital foramen and on to the front of the maxilla.

If you look into the pterygomaxillary fissure from the side (Figs 10.1 and 10.3) you will see a round

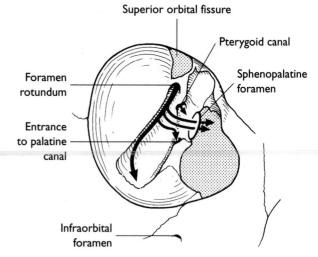

Figure 10.4 Branches of the maxillary nerve passing through the foramen rotundum into the pterygopalatine fossa run either forwards in the infraorbital fissure and canal toward the infraorbital foramen, medially through the sphenopalatine foramen into the nose and roof of the pharynx, or downwards in the palatine canal to the palate. Autonomic nerves emerging from the pterygoid canal also run forwards into the pterygopalatine fossa and join with all these nerves.

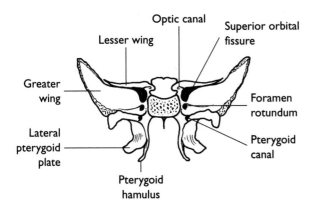

Figure 10.5 A disarticulated sphenoid bone seen from behind. The superior orbital fissure separates the lesser and greater wings of the sphenoid. The foramen rotundum and pterygoid canal run directly forwards through the body of the sphenoid to open into the pterygopalatine fossa. Note that the medial pterygoid plate has a hamulus around which the tendon of tensor palati runs into the soft palate.

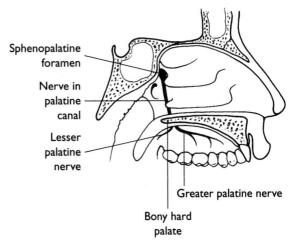

Figure 10.6 Sensory nerves destined for the palate run from the pterygopalatine fossa and into the palatine canal in the lateral wall of the nose. They emerge at the lesser and greater palatine foramina on the hard palate.

foramen deep within the pterygopalatine fossa. This leads further inwards to the lateral wall and roof of the nose. It is called the **sphenopalatine foramen**, so named because part of both the sphenoid and the palatine bone contribute to it.

Finally, look at the bony palate that forms the roof of the mouth (Fig. 10.6). Another canal runs from the pterygopalatine fossa down into the side of the hard palate. This is the **palatine canal**. It eventually divides to open as two foramina, the greater and lesser palatine foramina on the hard palate. These lie opposite the last molar tooth on the hard palate where the palatine bone sutures with the maxilla.

Figure 10.7 shows how the nerves that run through this region relate to these foramina and to the bony canals that run into and out of the pterygopalatine fossa. The large maxillary division of the trigeminal nerve (Vii) leaves the skull through the foramen rotundum and then enters the infraorbital canal to emerge at the infraorbital foramen. While in the pterygopalatine fossa several branches of this important nerve either diverge medially into the nose through the sphenopalatine foramen, or forwards through the orbit, or downwards towards the palate through the bony canals just described. Note also the **pterygoid canal** of the sphenoid bone which transmits autonomic nerves to the pterygopalatine fossa. The pterygopalatine fossa contains many nerves and blood vessels and is an important point of relay for nerves and vessels in the nose and mid-face.

The bones of the nasal cavity

The **nasal bones** lie in front of the maxilla (Fig. 10.8) and form the bridge of the nose. Recall again the position of the ethmoid bone in between the orbital cavities and also the position of the **lacrimal bone** and the **nasolacrimal canal**. This contains the **naso-lacrimal duct** which runs from the orbit to the floor of the nose. Figure 10.8 is of the bones that form the lateral walls of the nose. The structures of the roof and floor can also be seen in the diagram. Notice that the roof of the nose is formed by the ethmoid bone in front and the sphenoid bone behind. The body of the sphenoid contains the sphenoidal air sinus. In front, the floor and lateral wall of the nose is formed by the maxilla and behind by the palatine bone. When viewed from the front, this latter bone is shaped like a letter 'L'. It takes part in both the formation of the floor of the nose (hard palate) and of the lateral wall of the nose. The vertical part of the bone is forked at the top (Fig. 10.3) and makes up the lower part of the sphenopalatine foramen. Understand from Figure 10.8 how the maxillary air sinus lies in front of the pterygopalatine fossa. The sphenopalatine foramen, leading from the fossa into the nose, is indicated by the arrow. It passes between the fork at the top of the perpendicular plate of the palatine bone. The lateral wall of the nose is easier to understand. The maxilla forms a large part of the lateral wall of the nasal cavity. In it is an opening from the maxillary air sinus

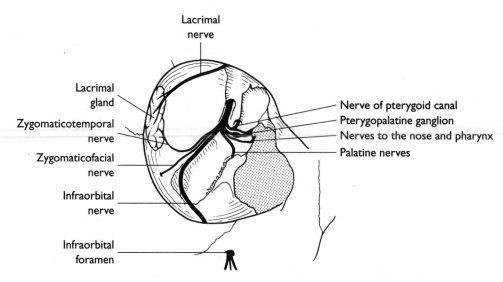

Figure 10.7   Branches of the zygomatic nerve communicate with the lacrimal nerve on the lateral wall of the orbital cavity and also pierce the zygomatic bone to supply the skin over the side of the cheek. Branches of the maxillary nerve run: (i) from the foramen rotundum to the front of the cheek; (ii) to the pharynx; (iii) to the lateral wall of the nose; and (iv) to the palate. The nerve of the pterygoid canal runs forwards to the pterygomandibular ganglion which is suspended from the maxillary nerve.

into the nasal cavity. Above this opening, the lateral wall is formed by the ethmoid bone.

This is a good time to look at the ethmoid bone in more detail (Fig. 10.9). The cribriform plate forms the roof of the nose and floor of the anterior cranial fossa. It has a midline projection called the crista galli. A downward extension of this, the **perpendicular plate** of the ethmoid, forms part of the midline nasal septum. On either side the bone is expanded by numerous air cells whose lateral walls lie in the medial walls of the orbital cavities. The ethmoid air cells also expand into the top of the nasal cavity to form **anterior, middle** and

posterior groups of **ethmoidal air cells** or **sinuses**.

The bony processes in the nasal cavity that curl over the air sinuses in the lateral wall of the nose are called **conchae**. There are three conchae. The superior and middle conchae are part of the ethmoid bone. The **inferior concha** is a separate bone. Beneath each concha there is a **meatus** or pocket.

Briefly turn your attention to the bones that form the midline nasal septum (Fig. 10.10) and be clear to distinguish this in your mind from the lateral wall of the nose. Above is the perpendicular plate of the

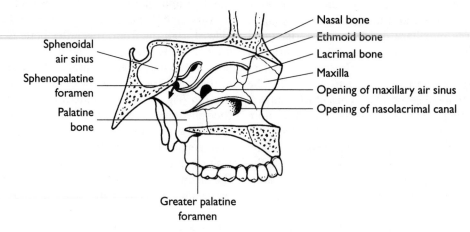

Figure 10.8   The bones of the roof, floor and lateral wall of the nose.

(a)

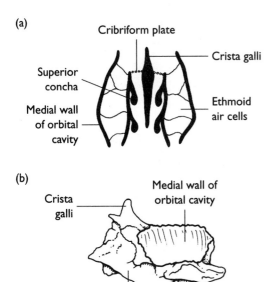

(b)

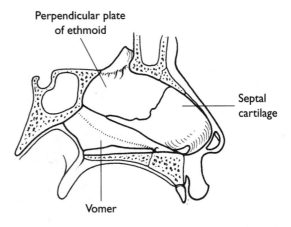

Figure 10.10 The midline septum of the nose is made up of the perpendicular plate of the ethmoid, the vomer and the septal cartilage.

Figure 10.9 The ethmoid bone in coronal section (a) and as seen laterally when disarticulated (b).

ethmoid; below is a thin flat bone called the **vomer**, which extends from behind like a wedge between the cranial base and the floor of the nose. The midline septum continues anteriorly as a cartilaginous **septal cartilage**.

The paranasal air sinuses

All the paranasal air sinuses are lined with respiratory mucous membrane. They all have a sensory nerve supply and a rich blood supply. Each one opens into the cavity of the nose. The maxillary air sinus is particularly important clinically and needs special attention. It is pyramidal in shape, the base being the lateral wall of the nose. The apex of the maxillary sinus lies close to the zygomatic bone. The roof consists of the floor of the orbit and the infraorbital canal lies in the roof. The anterior wall of the maxillary sinus lies behind the cheek. Behind the posterior wall lies the pterygomaxillary fissure and the pterygopalatine fossa. In the floor of the maxillary sinus the tips of the roots of several teeth create irregular bumps. These tooth roots are embedded in the **alveolar bone** of the maxilla. The maxillary air sinus sometimes

becomes infected. Then the respiratory mucous membrane swells and fluid may collect in the cavity, which can be painful (especially when bending forwards) in the face or even in the top teeth. The **ostium**, or hole, through which the maxillary sinus drains is high on the lateral wall of the nose beneath the middle concha at the front of a groove called the **hiatus semilunaris** (Fig. 10.11). This hiatus runs around the base of a swelling formed by a bulging of some of the ethmoidal air cells. The swelling protrudes a little into the middle meatus and is called the **bulla ethmoidalis**.

The air cells of the ethmoid bone drain into the cavity of the nose through holes which open under the middle and superior meati. The **sphenoidal air sinuses** drain into the nose through two openings high in the roof of the nose at the back, in a region called the **sphenoethmoidal recess**. Each frontal bone also contains an air sinus lateral to the midline. Sometimes there is a common sinus and occasionally one or other sinus will be absent. The **frontal sinus** drains into the nose on either side through a funnel-like opening called the **infundibulum**. This empties into the front of the hiatus semilunaris. The only structure to empty into the inferior meatus is the **nasolacrimal duct**. Notice the positions of openings into the lateral wall of the nose from each of the sinuses and the nasolacrimal duct (Fig. 10.11). Notice in particular the arrangement under the middle concha and also the opening of the auditory tube which lies at the level of the floor of the nose.

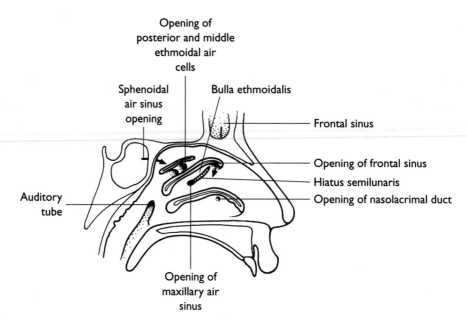

Figure 10.11 The conchae, or turbinate bones, have been cut away from the lateral wall of the nose. The openings of the air sinuses, nasolacrimal duct and auditory tube are indicated.

Nerves in the nose and midface

The trigeminal nerve (the Vth cranial nerve) is a mixed cranial nerve. It is the largest of the cranial nerves. The trigeminal nerve has a large ganglion which contains the cell bodies of its sensory fibres. This lies just within the middle cranial fossa, in a depression on the apex of the petrous temporal bone. As the nerve grows forwards during development, it pushes underneath the dura mater of the middle cranial fossa for a short distance before the dura eventually fuses around it. In so doing it draws its covering of arachnoid mater with it up to the point of fusion. The first part of the nerve and its sensory ganglion, therefore, are bathed in cerebrospinal fluid in a subarachnoid space that lies beneath the dura of the middle cranial fossa. This space is called **Meckel's cave**. Beyond the ganglion the trigeminal nerve divides into three great divisions on the floor of the middle cranial fossa. The **ophthalmic division** (Vi) passes forwards through the superior orbital fissure into the orbit; we have already studied its branches. The second division is the **maxillary nerve** (Vii). This passes forwards through the foramen rotundum into the pterygopalatine fossa. The **mandibular division** (Viii) is the only division with motor fibres and it immediately passes directly downwards through an

oval foramen in the skull base that we know is called the foramen ovale.

The maxillary division leaves the skull through the foramen rotundum and enters the pterygopalatine fossa. Here it divides into several branches (Fig. 10.7). The **zygomatic** nerve passes along the lateral wall of the orbital cavity and its branches run through the zygomatic bone to supply the skin overlying this bone and the skin over the temple. The **infraorbital** nerve runs forwards through the infraorbital canal to emerge deep in the cheek (Fig. 10.12). It supplies sensation to the lower eyelid and conjunctiva, the skin of the mid-face and upper lip. The **nasopalatine** branch of the maxillary nerve passes medially through the sphenopalatine foramen and into the roof and lateral wall of the nose (Fig. 10.7). Another branch of the maxillary nerve runs down from the pterygopalatine fossa to supply sensation to the palate. The palatine nerves open into the palate via the greater and lesser palatine foramina (Fig. 10.6).

While still in the pterygopalatine fossa the maxillary nerve gives off **posterior superior alveolar nerves**. These run into the back of the maxillary tuberosity and on through the bone to form a plexus over the tips of the roots of the upper molar teeth in the floor of the antrum (Fig. 10.12). **Middle superior alveolar nerves** branch off the infraorbital nerve in

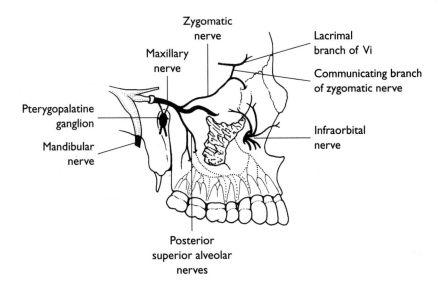

Figure 10.12   The maxillary nerve seen in lateral view. Branches of the zygomatic nerve supply skin over the temple and zygomatic bone and some communicate with branches of the lacrimal nerve. The posterior superior alveolar nerves enter the maxillary tuberosity and form a plexus with other superior alveolar nerves in the floor of the maxillary antrum. (After Basmajian JV and Slonecker CE (1989) *Grant's Method of Anatomy*, 11th edn. Baltimore: Williams and Wilkins.)

the roof of the maxillary antrum and also run into the plexus, sometimes as far forwards as the canine tooth in the floor of the antrum. The **anterior superior alveolar nerve** (Fig. 10.13) is another branch of the infraorbital nerve. It runs to the incisor and canine teeth in the bone behind the margin of the nasal aperture. In this way all the upper teeth are supplied by the maxillary division of the trigeminal nerve. The anterior superior alveolar nerve is especially important because it also gives some branches that supply sensation to part of the front of the lateral wall of the nose, the floor of the nose, as well as the front of the midline septum of the nose.

Autonomic nerves in the nose and mid-face

In the head, we always find parasympathetic ganglia near terminal branches of the trigeminal nerve. We described the **ciliary ganglion** in the orbit previously, close to the **nasociliary branch** of the ophthalmic division of the trigeminal nerve. Similarly, another ganglion called the **pterygopalatine ganglion** lies in the pterygopalatine fossa. Here, it is connected to the maxillary division of the trigeminal nerve (Figs 10.7 and 10.12). Like the other parasympathetic

ganglia in the head, the pterygopalatine ganglion is a relay station for the parasympathetic neurons of the region. Actually, these neurons do not leave the brain in the trigeminal nerve but in the facial nerve (the VIIth crainal nerve). Recall for a moment the passage of the facial nerve through its canal in the petrous temporal bone (look back to Figure 3.12). Parasympathetic neurons destined for the pterygopalatine ganglion leave the facial nerve in the larger of the two **petrosal nerves**. This **greater superficial petrosal nerve** passes from a slit on the

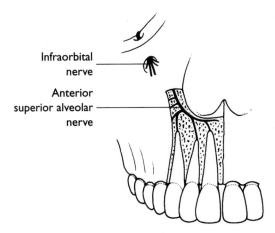

Figure 10.13   The anterior superior alveolar nerve runs within the bone of the maxilla just lateral to the bony nasal margin. It supplies the upper anterior teeth with sensation.

front of the petrous temporal bone into the pterygoid canal of the sphenoid bone. The nerve runs through the canal and carries the parasympathetic neurons into the pterygopalatine fossa. Here they enter the pterygopalatine ganglion suspended from the maxillary nerve. They synapse in the ganglion and postganglionic nerve fibres are distributed through all the sensory branches of the maxillary nerve to their target glands. Parasympathetic motor nerve fibres cause secretion of both mucous and serous glands in the nose, paranasal air sinuses and palate as well as secretion of tears by the lacrimal gland. Their action is said to mimic the symptoms of hay fever and this is a way to remember what they do.

Some postganglionic parasympathetic neurons pass directly from the pterygopalatine ganglion to the lacrimal gland. They do this by running up through the inferior orbital fissure and onto the posterolateral wall of the orbital cavity. From here they run forwards into the lacrimal gland and are secretomotor to it.

Like the other parasympathetic ganglia, the pterygopalatine ganglion also has other neurons passing through it. These do not synapse but simply pass through on their way to target organs. These include sympathetic neurons which have climbed up the internal carotid artery and which have also then entered the pterygoid canal in the back of the sphenoid bone. As they approach the canal these sympathetic nerve fibres are called collectively the **deep petrosal nerve.** They pass through the pterygoid canal in company with the parasympathetic neurons and arrive at the pterygopalatine fossa. Once here, sympathetic fibres pass straight through the pterygopalatine ganglion and distribute to the so-called glands of 'hay fever'. Generally they are vasoconstrictor in action. Within the pterygoid canal parasympathetic and sympathetic neurons pass along it side by side. All of these autonomic nerves are referred to collectively here as **the nerve of the pterygoid canal.**

Each of the major sensory nerve branches that arise from the maxillary nerve in the pterygopalatine fossa distribute both sympathetic and parasympathetic nerve fibres with them. The **nasopalatine nerve** passes through the sphenopalatine foramen into the nose. Branches of this cross the roof of the nose to get to the septum and then down to the anterior part of the hard palate (Fig. 10.14). **Lateral nasal** branches pass into the lateral wall of the nose from the pterygopalatine fossa. **Palatine nerves** pass down through

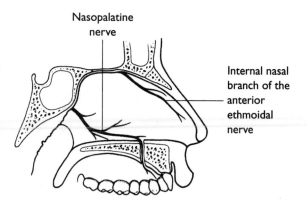

Figure 10.14   The nasopalatine nerve runs from the sphenopalatine foramen over the roof of the nose to the midline, descends on the midline nasal septum and runs finally through the incisive foramen. The internal branch of the anterior ethmoidal nerve runs into the front of the nasal septum above. These nerves are general sensory nerves, but autonomic nerve fibres also distribute with the nasopalatine nerve from the pterygopalatine ganglion.

the palatine canals towards the back of the hard palate. These palatine nerves also give off extra lateral nasal branches to the lateral wall of the nose on the way down (Fig. 10.15).

Two additional nerves need to be mentioned with respect to the structures of the nose we have described. One of these is the **anterior ethmoidal nerve** and the other is the **olfactory nerve** or first cranial nerve. It is sufficient to say that the anterior ethmoidal nerves are branches of the nasociliary nerve in the orbit. They leave the orbit through its medial wall and enter the anterior cranial fossa. From here they enter the nose through the sides of the cribriform plate of the ethmoid bone. They carry sensory impulses from the upper anterior segment of the nasal walls and the skin on bridge of the nose. The olfactory nerve rootlets carry the special sensations of smell from special receptors located in the upper part of the nasal septum, lateral wall and roof of the nose. These nerves pass through the cribriform plate of the ethmoid bone to reach the olfactory bulb which overlies it.

Blood supply to the nose

Each of the nerves we have described that pass either into the lateral wall of the nose or on to the roof of the nose or on to the midline nasal septum is accompanied by an artery. Many of these arteries

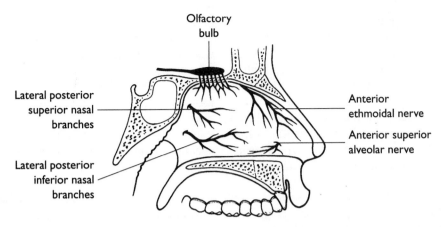

Figure 10.15 The mucous membrane of the lateral wall of the nose receives sensory fibres from: (i) lateral nasal branches posteriorly; (ii) anterior ethmoidal; and (iii) anterior superior alveolar nerves. Specialized olfactory epithelium covers the roof and upper part of the nasal cavity.

are branches of the maxillary artery, which has a complicated course into the pterygopalatine fossa. From here branches of the maxillary artery pass through the sphenopalatine foramen and become the **lateral nasal arteries** and **sphenopalatine artery**. There are also important contributions to the blood supply to the mucous membrane of the lateral wall of the nose from the **anterior ethmoidal artery** superiorly and from the **anterior superior alveolar artery** inferiorly. Oddly, it may seem, there is a significant contribution to the blood supply to the nasal septum from an ascending branch of the greater palatine artery which enters the nose through the incisive canal at the front of the hard palate (Fig. 10.16).

Applied anatomy of the nose

Sinusitis is a complication that usually follows a common cold or upper respiratory tract infection. Cilia of the respiratory epithelium within the sinuses cease to function effectively and the mucous membrane engorges and is inflamed. Drainage through the ostium of each sinus slows and is ineffective so that fluid accumulates within the cavity of the sinus. Maxillary sinusitis and frontal sinusitis are very common and present with pain on bending the head forwards. The mucosa around the ostium is the most sensitive area of each sinus. The maxillary sinus begins to form after birth. As the face grows,

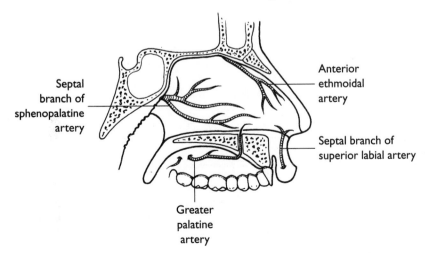

Figure 10.16 Arteries supplying the midline nasal septum anastomose with each other towards the front at a rich vascular plexus called Little's area.

epithelium is drawn into the body of the maxilla from the nose at a point that represents the opening of the ostium. The ostium remains high on the wall of the maxillary sinus in this original position, even when the face grows in height and the cavity of the sinus extends inferiorly. The result in the adult is a disadvantageous drainage point high on the medial wall of the maxillary sinus. One advantage to this is that secretions from the nasolacrimal duct, which opens into the inferior meatus, cannot then run into the maxillary antrum.

Epistaxis or nosebleeds can be very serious even though they are mostly of little consequence. The nasal mucous membrane has a rich blood supply and is erectile in nature. Alternate vasodilatation and vasoconstriction of the mucous membrane lining each nostril means that we often breathe through one side of the nose only for periods of time. It is a function of the nose to warm and humidify inspired air in this way and it is highly likely that the nasal mucous membrane is also involved in heat loss when core temperatures rise above 37°C. For these reasons the nasal mucous membrane is highly vascular. Nose bleeds may originate from a vascular plexus on either side of the nasal septum about 1.5 cm from the opening of the nostril. This region is called **Little's area.** It is here that many arteries anastomose on the septum (Fig. 10.16). They include branches of the superior labial artery, anterior ethmoidal artery, sphenopalatine artery and anterior superior alveolar artery. Nose bleeds that occur higher and further back in the nose can be serious and very difficult to stop. They are more common in older people with raised blood pressure (hypertension).

chapter 11

The Infratemporal and Temporal Fossae

The **mandible**, or lower jaw, has two **mandibular condyles** that articulate with the left and right temporal bones at the **temporomandibular joints** (Fig. 11.1). The **body** of the mandible lies on either side of the mouth and is continuous at the **mandibular symphysis** in the midline anteriorly. The **ascending ramus** of the mandible runs between the posterior aspect of the body and the condyle above. The point on the lower border of the mandible at which the body and the ascending ramus are continuous is called the **angle** of the mandible. Anteriorly, the ascending ramus is surmounted by a **coronoid process.** There is a **mandibular notch** between the coronoid process and the condyle in the upper border of the ascending ramus.

The structures within the **temporal** and **infra-** temporal fossae lie between the pharynx and the side of the face. The **infratemporal fossa** lies between the pharynx and the ascending ramus of the mandible. The roof of the fossa is the base of the skull. Much of this roof is formed by the undersurface of the greater wing of the sphenoid bone. Look at Figure 5.2 again and identify the foramen ovale and the foramen spinosum that pass through the sphenoid bone in this region. Notice also the position of the **stylomastoid foramen** in the temporal bone, just deep to the **mastoid process** and lateral to the **styloid process.** Understand that the styloid process of the temporal bone and the **tympanic plate** of the temporal bone lie towards the back of the roof of the infratemporal fossa and that the pterygoid plates of the sphenoid bone lie in front.

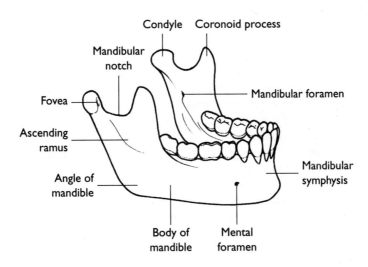

Figure 11.1 The mandible and its major bony landmarks.

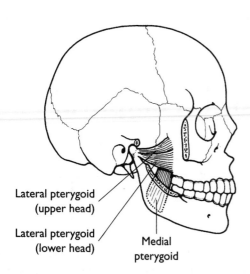

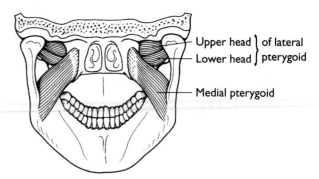

Figure 11.3 The lateral pterygoid runs anteroposteriorly and passes laterally from the lateral aspects of the lateral pterygoid plates to the condyles and discs. The medial pterygoid runs superoinferiorly, in the same direction as the masseter, but on the inner aspect of the mandible.

Figure 11.2 The lateral pterygoid muscle arises as two heads (an upper and a lower head) and inserts into both the fovea of the neck of the mandible and articular disc of the TMJ. The medial pterygoid arises from the medial aspect of the lateral pterygoid plate and inserts into the mandible at the angle.

The muscles of mastication

There are four large muscles attached to the ascending ramus and condyle of the mandible. These move the mandible during chewing, speaking and swallowing. They are called collectively the muscles of mastication. Two of these muscles attach to the outside and two to the inside of the mandible. The two on the inside are called the **medial pterygoid** muscle and the **lateral pterygoid** muscle and the two on the outside are the **masseter** and **temporalis** muscles.

The lateral pterygoid muscle (Fig. 11.2) arises from the undersurface of the greater wing of the sphenoid bone and the lateral aspect of the lateral pterygoid plate of the sphenoid bone. These two surfaces are continuous and next to each other; they are simply the roof of the infratemporal fossa that faces downwards and medial wall of the infratemporal fossa that faces laterally. The lateral pterygoid muscle arises as two heads, an upper and a lower head, one from each of these surfaces of the sphenoid bone. There are structures that squeeze between these two heads on their way in and out of the infratemporal fossa. Most of the lateral pterygoid muscle inserts into the neck of the mandible just below the condyle, into a depression here called the **fovea** (Fig. 11.1). Notice

that the muscle runs backwards and laterally from its origin in order to do this. A part of the upper head inserts into the **disc** or **meniscus** of the temporomandibular joint. The lateral pterygoid muscle is active when we protrude our chin or open our mouths. The upper head is also active on closing the mouth. It steadies the meniscus and condylar head against the posterior slope of the articular eminence as they slide back into the glenoid fossa. We will study this muscle and its actions further when we describe the temporomandibular joint.

The medial pterygoid muscle (Fig. 11.3) arises from the medial aspect of the lateral pterygoid plate and inserts into the inner aspect of the angle of the mandible. This muscle runs downwards and laterally to reach the lower margin of the ascending ramus. The medial pterygoid muscle is active during closure of the jaws as when biting or occluding the teeth together.

The masseter muscle (Fig. 11.4) takes origin from the zygomatic arch and also runs downwards. The masseter has two parts to it. The deeper part takes origin from the inner surface of the zygomatic arch and runs vertically down to the outer aspect of the ramus. The superficial part takes origin further anteriorly from the undersurface of the zygomatic arch. This part runs downwards and backwards to the outer surface of the ascending ramus of the mandible. The masseter muscle closes the mandible and occludes the teeth together.

The temporalis muscle (Fig. 11.4) arises from the side of the vault of the skull and from a tough fascia that covers the surface of the muscle called the

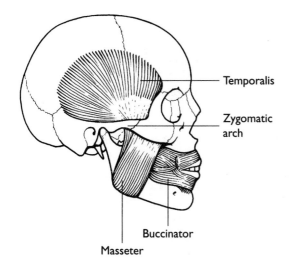

Figure 11.4 Temporalis arises from the vault of the skull and converges as a tendon on to the coronoid process and ascending ramus of the mandible. The masseter has a deep head which is mostly covered by a larger part, the superficial head. Both run between the ascending ramus and angle of the mandible and the zygomatic bone.

temporalis fascia. The side of the vault bones are marked with **temporal lines** where the muscle takes origin from the bone. The temporalis muscle passes through the **temporal fossa.** This fossa is bounded laterally by the zygomatic arch. The temporalis muscle inserts on to the **coronoid process** of the mandible and inner aspect of the anterior border of the ascending ramus. Temporalis is yet another muscle that occludes the teeth and is active during jaw closure.

Chewing is actually a very complicated process. Many of the muscles of mastication are active at different times during the chewing cycle. Chewing involves an alternating pattern of lateral mandibular movements which shift the mandible from left to right as well as simply grinding the teeth on one side together. The masseter and the pterygoids play an important role in this lateral movement of the mandible at the same time as they bring about movements of jaw closure and opening. Speech and swallowing are a little different. Movements of the mandible are only ever up and down during speech. Always during swallowing solids there is firm bilateral occlusion of the jaws while the tongue forces food backwards into the oropharynx.

Nerves in the infratemporal fossa

Two nerves pass through the skull base and into the infratemporal fossa. They are the mandibular division of the trigeminal nerve (Vii) and the facial nerve (the VIIth cranial nerve). The mandibular nerve leaves through the foramen ovale and carries both motor and sensory fibres to the infratemporal fossa and mouth. The facial nerve carries motor fibres to the superficial muscles of the face. Besides the muscles that move the mandible, and the facial and mandibular nerves, there are other structures in the infratemporal fossa. Towards the back of the infratemporal fossa there is a group of structures that run through the neck. These include the internal carotid artery and jugular vein as well as cranial nerves IX, X, XI and XII. One of the terminal branches of the external carotid artery, the maxillary artery, runs a complicated course through the infratemporal fossa. Finally, the **parotid gland,** a large salivary gland, lies behind the ascending ramus of the mandible and extends medially into the infratemporal fossa. During its development the parotid gland grows out from the oral cavity and back into the structures of the neck and face behind the mandible.

The mandibular division of the trigeminal nerve (Viii) drops vertically down through the foramen ovale in the base of the skull to reach the infratemporal fossa (Fig. 11.5). Unlike the other two divisions of the trigeminal nerve, the mandibular nerve contains both sensory and motor neurons. In the infratemporal fossa the nerve finds itself deep to the lateral pterygoid muscle and on the surface of the tensor palati muscle. At this point it gives off a tiny branch containing sensory neurons which follows the middle meningeal artery through the foramen spinosum into the skull. This carries sensation from part of the middle cranial fossa and the mastoid air cells. The mandibular nerve has a parasympathetic ganglion suspended from beneath it just below the foramen ovale. This is the **otic ganglion** and it contains synapses between preganglionic and postganglionic parasympathetic nerve fibres destined for the parotid gland. It also has sympathetic neurons running through it which do not synapse within it.

The mandibular nerve divides into anterior and posterior divisions. All the branches of the **anterior division**, except one, are motor to the muscles of mastication and to a muscle of the soft palate.

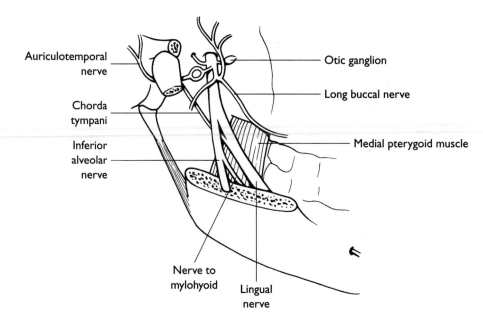

Auriculotemporal nerve

Chorda tympani

Inferior alveolar nerve

Nerve to mylohyoid

Lingual nerve

Otic ganglion

Long buccal nerve

Medial pterygoid muscle

Figure 11.5   The mandibular division of the trigeminal nerve and its major branches in the infratemporal fossa.

Branches from this division therefore go to the medial and lateral pterygoids, and to the temporalis and masseter muscles. The masseter is supplied by a branch from the anterior division which gets to the muscle by passing through the notch between the condyle and coronoid process of the mandible. In addition the anterior division of the mandibular nerve supplies the tensor palati muscle on which the nerve lies beneath the foramen ovale. The only sensory branch of the anterior division is the **long buccal nerve** which carries sensation from the inside and outside of the cheek. This nerve runs back from the cheek between the two heads of the lateral pterygoid muscle to join the anterior division high in the infratemporal fossa.

In contrast, the **posterior division** is primarily made up of sensory nerve fibres. It has two large and important branches, the **lingual nerve** and the **inferior alveolar nerve**. Both of these lie on the lateral surface of the medial pterygoid muscle in the infratemporal fossa. The lingual nerve is destined for the tongue and the inferior alveolar nerve for the lower teeth, lower lip and chin. A third branch of this division is the **auriculotemporal nerve** which carries sensation from the temple and auricle. We will look at these three branches in some detail since their functions are important.

The inferior alveolar nerve passes down over the lateral surface of the medial pterygoid muscle towards the **mandibular foramen** on the inside of the mandible.

Here it enters the bone of the mandible and passes forwards beneath the lower teeth supplying them. It leaves the front of the mandible through another foramen called the **mental foramen**. The **mental nerve** carries sensation from the skin of the lower lip and the point of the chin. Before entering the mandibular foramen the inferior alveolar nerve gives off a motor branch. This is the only motor branch of the posterior division. It runs to two muscles in the floor of the mouth, it is **the nerve to the mylohyoid** and **anterior belly of the digastric.**

The lingual nerve is joined by the **chorda tympani** under the base of the skull. This is a branch of the VIIth cranial nerve that we last mentioned when we studied the middle ear cavity. Look once again at the branches of the VIIth cranial nerve in the petrous temporal bone in Figures 3.4 and 3.11. The chorda tympani is seen coursing through the middle ear. It leaves the floor of this cavity through the **petrotympanic fissure**. This fissure opens very close to the spine of the sphenoid bone on the cranial base which in turn is very close to the foramen ovale (Fig. 10.1). The chorda tympani has only a little distance to travel at this point before it is able to join the lingual nerve. The chorda tympani is one of the two parasympathetic nerve bundles of the VIIth nerve. We described the greater superficial petrosal branch as going to the pterygopalatine ganglion. The chorda tympani aims for the infratemporal fossa. The chorda

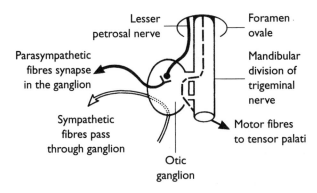

Figure 11.6 The mandibular division of the trigeminal nerve and the lesser superficial petrosal nerve pass through the foramen ovale. The otic ganglion is suspended below the foramen ovale and contains synapses between the preganglionic and postganglionic parasympathetic fibres destined for the parotid gland. Other fibres, however, pass through the ganglion without synapsing.

tympani carries parasympathetic fibres which 'hitch-hike' down the lingual nerve to supply the salivary glands and mucous glands of the floor of the mouth. It also carries taste fibres in the opposite direction from the anterior two-thirds of the tongue to the brain.

The auriculotemporal nerve is the third important sensory branch of the posterior division of the mandibular nerve. The nerve has **two roots** which embrace the **middle meningeal artery**. It then passes laterally to supply sensation to part of the ear, tympanic membrane and temple. At its origin it is in close relationship to the otic ganglion.

Parasympathetic neurons destined for the otic ganglion arise from the glossopharyngeal nerve (the IXth cranial nerve). These fibres leave the glossopharyngeal nerve just below the jugular foramen. They then pass up through the petrous temporal bone and middle ear cavity and leave it again through its anterior surface as the **lesser superficial petrosal nerve**. The lesser petrosal nerve drops down through the foramen ovale in company with the mandibular division of the trigeminal nerve (Fig. 11.6). It is then perfectly situated to enter the otic ganglion and synapse within it. From the ganglion, postganglionic parasympathetic neurons jump into the auriculotemporal nerve. They run in this nerve to the side of the mandible where they leave to enter the large parotid salivary gland which lies in this position. They bring about secretion of saliva from the parotid gland. As with all the parasympathetic ganglia in the head, sympathetic neurons also pass through the otic ganglion but do

not synapse within it. They too run on to the parotid gland.

The maxillary and superficial temporal arteries

As the external carotid artery approaches the infratemporal fossa it divides into its two terminal branches. These are the **maxillary** and **superficial temporal arteries** (Fig. 11.7). The maxillary artery passes in a tortuous fashion through the infratemporal fossa. It usually passes between the two heads of the lateral pterygoid muscle to enter the pterygopalatine fossa. The artery has many branches in both the infratemporal and in the pterygopalatine fossae. These supply the ear, nose, palate and pharynx. However, there is no merit whatever in trying to learn the names of all the branches. Basically, the branches of the outer third of the artery go into bony structures such as the middle ear, the maxilla and the mandible. The branches from the middle third of the artery go to each of the muscles of mastication. The innermost third of the artery we have already studied in the context of the nose. These branches arise near the sphenopalatine foramen and for the most part again travel into bony structures and canals to reach their destination.

Note only one or two important branches at this point. The **inferior alveolar artery** accompanies the nerve of the same name into the mandible and through to the chin as the **mental artery**. It supplies the pulps of the teeth and the body of the mandible with blood. The **middle meningeal artery** is important. It is a nutrient artery for the bones of the vault of the skull. The vessel ascends through the foramen spinosum. In its ascent it is embraced by the two roots of the auriculotemporal nerve. It gains the interval between the dura and periosteum of the skull. An accessory meningeal artery ascends through the foramen ovale and, among other things, helps to supply the ganglion of the trigeminal nerve. Branches of the maxillary artery supply the external acoustic meatus and tympanic membrane.

Muscular branches also follow branches of the mandibular nerve and supply all the muscles of mastication. Finally, in the pterygopalatine fossa, branches follow each of the branches of the pterygopalatine ganglion. One important artery follows the infraorbital

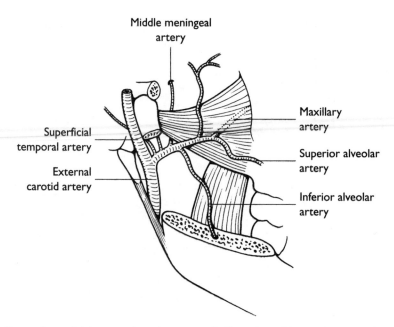

Figure 11.7 The maxillary and superficial temporal arteries are terminal branches of the external carotid artery in the infratemporal fossa. The first few branches of the maxillary artery enter bony structures associated with the infratemporal fossa.

nerve and emerges with it on to the cheek through the infraorbital foramen.

The pterygoid plexus of veins

A network of veins lies around the pterygoid muscles. This is the **pterygoid venous plexus**. The plexus receives blood from veins which accompany the local arteries. It also receives blood from the inferior orbital veins through the inferior orbital fissure. Eventually, the plexus drains into a pair of **short maxillary veins** which lie deep to the neck of the mandible. These join the **superficial temporal vein** to form the **retromandibular vein** (Fig. 11.8). It has a few important connections. A **deep facial vein** connects the plexus with the facial vein. Another connection is through the foramen ovale to the cavernous sinus. This is an important connection since infection, for example from an upper wisdom tooth, can track up this path if unchecked. More commonly, local anaesthetic given to block the posterior superior alveolar nerves at the back of the maxilla can easily be misplaced into the pterygoid plexus of veins from where it may drain into the cavernous sinus. When we yawn we squeeze venous blood out of the pterygoid plexus. Large amounts of local anaesthetic can there-fore very easily find their way into the cavernous sinus. The effect may be a transient anaesthesia of the VIth cranial nerve, the abducens, which, as you will remember, is the only cranial nerve in the cavern-ous sinus to run free in the venous blood beneath the carotid artery. The other cranial nerves run in the dura of the wall of the sinus and are thus more protected from the effects of local anaesthetic in the venous blood. So, should a patient having upper wisdom teeth removed ever complain of seeing double, it is wise to test the abducent nerve and reassure them it will recover.

The posterior part of the infratemporal fossa con-tains the internal carotid artery and internal jugular vein. They each run to their respective foramina in the base of the skull. Also leaving the skull in this region are the IXth, Xth, XIth and XIIth cranial nerves. Superimposed upon and between these struc-tures is the styloid process and its muscles.

The temporomandibular joint

The **temporomandibular joint** (or TMJ) is a synovial articulation between the **glenoid fossa** on the under-surface of the temporal bone and the **condyle** or **head** of the mandible (Fig. 11.9). It has a fibrous

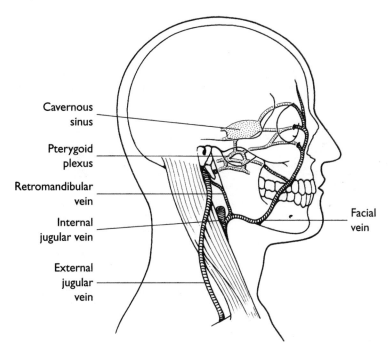

Cavernous sinus

Pterygoid plexus

Retromandibular vein

Internal jugular vein

External jugular vein

Facial vein

Figure 11.8   The veins of the face and of the pterygoid plexus of veins that weave through each lateral pterygoid muscle communicate with the cavernous venous sinuses intracranially.

capsule which is attached to the articular margins. The lateral part of the capsule is thickened to form a **lateral ligament**. The capsule is lined with synovial membrane. The joint cavity is completely divided into two by a disc of dense fibrous connective tissue. The disc is sometimes called the **meniscus**. The upper cavity of the joint is long and includes both a concave surface of the temporal bone and a convex bulge on the undersurface of the root of the zygomatic arch. This latter bulge is called the **articular eminence**. The upper chamber allows sliding of the head of the mandible forwards on to the eminence. During simple wide opening of the jaw the condyle slides forwards on to the eminence. The lower cavity has a simpler arrangement and allows hinge-like rotation during opening and closing of the mouth. However, it is likely that only the first millimetre or two of opening is entirely simple rotation in the lower joint compartment. The rest is a combination of both sliding and hinge movements. The capsule of the joint is also lax enough to allow small side-to-side movements to occur.

Two other ligaments attach to the mandible but are unlikely to limit movements of the joint to any great extent. The **sphenomandibular ligament** passes from the **spine** of the sphenoid bone on the base of

the skull to the **lingula**, a spur of bone that flanks the mandibular foramen (Fig. 11.10). This ligament is the remnant of the perichondrium of **Meckel's cartilage** of the first pharyngeal arch. The **stylomandibular ligament** arises from the styloid process and is attached to the angle of the mandible. It is a condensation of deep cervical investing fascia in the neck which spans two bony points.

When the mouth is opened the condyle and articular disc both move forwards and downwards on to the articular eminence of the temporal bone. At the same time the head of the condyle rotates on the lower surface of the disc. You can easily confirm this by palpating your own joint during wide opening and limited opening of the mouth. Protrusion occurs when both mandibular heads move anteriorly, together with their discs, as when sticking one's chin out. It is the lateral pterygoid muscle that pulls the condyles and discs forwards. Notice again how they run anteroposteriorly from origin to insertion. Notice how the medial pterygoids run superoinferiorly at right angles to this.

When we chew food we usually chew on one side for a while and then switch to the other in a rhythmic manner. This concentrates all the muscle force from both sides of the skull between the teeth of the

(a)

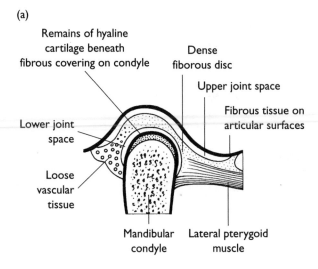

(b)

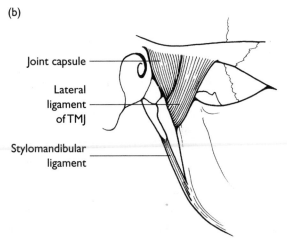

Figure 11.9 Sagittal section through the temporomandibular joint (a). A dense fibrous articular disc, or meniscus, separates the head of the condyle from the glenoid fossa of the temporal bone. Sliding movements of the condyle bring the condyle down on to the posterior aspect of the articular eminence during opening movements of the mandible. The lateral aspect of the joint (b) has a tough ligament which is attached to the neck of the mandible and to the zygomatic arch, and which helps to keep the condyle in the close packed position. The temporomandibular ligament overlies part of the joint capsule. (After Tonge CH and Luke DA (1979) The temporomandibular joint. *Dental Update* **6**: 213–217.)

chewing side. To chew on one side, the mandible swings over to that side so that the condyle of the opposite side then slides down on to the articular eminence. But on the chewing side, the condyle remains against the back of the eminence. This is why when patients fracture their condylar necks it

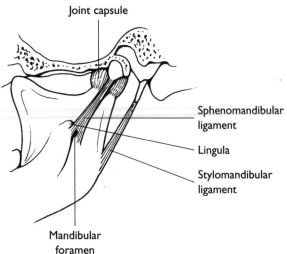

Figure 11.10 The stylomandibular and the sphenomandibular ligaments are embryological remnants and condensations of connective tissue. They have minimal, if any, limiting effects on mandibular movement.

hurts most when they try to chew on the *opposite* side.

The temporalis, masseter and medial pterygoid muscles act to close the mouth and occlude the teeth. As we noted previously, the upper head of the lateral pterygoid is also active during jaw closure since it steadies the disc while it returns to the glenoid fossa. Opening of the mouth against resistance is effected by the lower head of the lateral pterygoid and the digastric muscle.

The parotid gland

The **parotid gland** is a serous salivary gland. There are no mucous-secreting acini in the parotid. The parotid gland squeezes into the space available around the ramus of the mandible (Fig. 11.11). The part lying on the surface is called the **superficial lobe** and the deep tapering edge is called the **deep lobe**. Behind, it extends up to the neck of the mandible and this part is given the name of the **glenoid lobe** (Fig. 11.12). It is surrounded by the deep **investing fascia** of the neck. Swelling of the gland produces tension and considerable pain because of this complete envelope. This is why mumps (viral parotitis) is so painful. The superficial lobe extends forwards on to the surface of the masseter. The **parotid duct** emerges from its

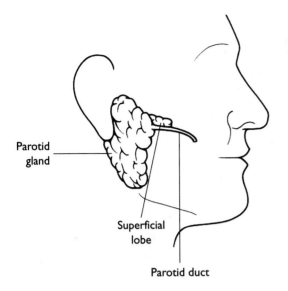

Parotid gland

Superficial lobe

Parotid duct

Figure 11.11 The parotid gland lies between the ear and the ascending ramus of the mandible. A superficial part of the parotid gland lies along the parotid duct on the surface of the masseter muscle. The duct itself runs over the masseter and pierces the buccinator to open into the mouth.

convex anterior edge. This pierces the cheek to enter the mouth somewhere near the second upper molar tooth at the level of its neck or cervix. If the duct opening were any lower in the cheek it would be prone to being chewed when we eat. The parotid gland has branches of the VIIth nerve embedded within it and these emerge from the anterior edge of the gland to pass to the facial musculature.

The glenoid lobe lies behind the temporomandibular joint in contact with the bony part of the external auditory meatus. It is also in close relationship to the auriculotemporal branch of the mandibular nerve here. Recall that this nerve is the final pathway for parasympathetic fibres to reach the gland. Remember also that parasympathetic neurons originate in the glossopharyngeal nerve (the XIth cranial nerve). They then leave the petrous temporal bone as the lesser petrosal nerve and drop down through the foramen ovale to synapse in the otic ganglion. Postganglionic parasympathetic neurons then jump into the auriculotemporal nerve. They promote secretion of saliva into the mouth when stimulated. Sympathetic fibres are also involved in secretor motor activity in the salivary glands and a balance of the different constituents of saliva results from this dual autonomic innervation. Volume of salivary flow over time depends in part upon the blood flow through the gland, and this is under vasomotor sympathetic control.

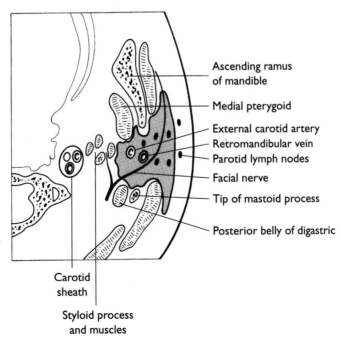

Ascending ramus of mandible

Medial pterygoid

External carotid artery
Retromandibular vein
Parotid lymph nodes

Facial nerve

Tip of mastoid process

Posterior belly of digastric

Carotid sheath

Styloid process and muscles

Figure 11.12 Transverse section through the neck just below the level of the skull base. The facial nerve, retromandibular vein and external carotid artery each run within the substance of the parotid duct. (After Tonge CH and Luke DA (1984) The salivary glands. *Dental Update* **11**: 264–270.)

Posteriorly, the gland is related to the mastoid process and to the sternocleidomastoid muscle (Fig. 11.12). The deep part of the gland is related to the styloid process and its muscles and to the internal carotid artery and internal jugular vein with their related cranial nerves. The external carotid artery, retromandibular vein and facial nerve pass through the substance of the gland. This makes removal of cysts or tumours from the parotid, for example, very difficult. Branches of the facial nerve have to be identified carefully and preserved during surgery. Note how the facial nerve is superficial in the parotid gland and how the retromandibular vein lies beneath it, and how the terminal branches of the external carotid artery lie deepest within the gland.

Before leaving the infratemporal fossa we can usefully consider the side of the mouth at this point. We need to describe the **buccinator muscle** (Fig. 11.13). Buccinator is technically a muscle of facial expression supplied by the facial nerve (the VIIth cranial nerve). It arises from the **pterygomandibular raphé** with superior constrictor posterior to this raphé. It runs forwards to the angle of the mouth and is attached above and below the molar and premolar teeth to the maxilla and the mandible for most of its course. Its upper and lower fibres cross as they approach the angle of the mouth. This is the point at which many muscles of facial expression intermingle and it is called the **modiolus**.

The important function of buccinator is to squeeze food from the cheek back between the teeth and into the mouth again for more chewing before being swallowed. To some extent it controls the flow of saliva through the parotid duct and prevents food and debris or air being squeezed back into the duct. It does this by contracting around the duct as the duct enters the mouth.

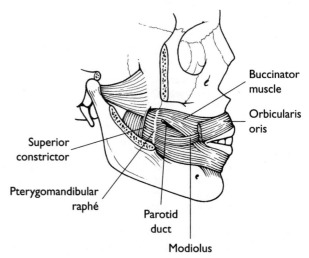

Figure 11.13   The superior constrictor and the buccinator meet at a seam, or pterygomandibular raphé, at the back of the cheek. Muscle fibres of the buccinator decussate at the modiolus at the corner of the mouth and are continuous there with the fibres of orbicularis oris. The parotid duct pierces the buccinator.

chapter 12

The Mouth and Face

The roof of the mouth

The front of the palate has a bony roof and is referred to as the **hard palate**, whereas behind it is entirely muscular and called the **soft palate**. The palate forms a partition between the mouth and the nose. The bony palate (Fig. 12.1) is bounded in front and at the sides by the two bony **alveolar processes** of the maxillae. The maxillary teeth lie in this ridge of supporting bone. The anterior two-thirds of the bony hard palate is formed by the **palatine processes of the maxillae**. The posterior one-third is made up of the two **horizontal plates** of the **palatine bones**. The bones are separated by a midline suture. The **greater palatine canal** divides as it approaches the

palate on its descent from the pterygopalatine fossa. One group of nerves and vessels passes into the palate just medial to the upper third molar tooth in the **palatine bone** at the **greater palatine foramen**. Another small group passes through the **lesser palatine foramen** just a short distance behind it. The **greater palatine nerves** and **vessels** run anteriorly along the sides of the hard palate in a groove. The **lesser palatine nerves** and **vessels** run posteriorly into the soft palate. Behind the incisor teeth is the **incisive fossa** and **canal** which conducts the terminal branches of the **nasopalatine nerve** into the front of the hard palate. Branches of the **greater palatine arteries** also pass up into the nose through this foramen for a short distance. The mucous

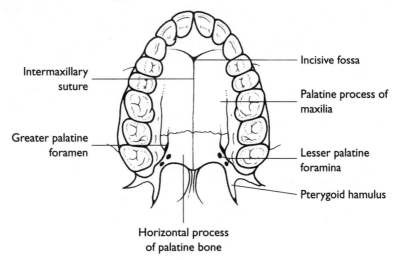

Intermaxillary suture

Greater palatine foramen

Horizontal process of palatine bone

Incisive fossa

Palatine process of maxilla

Lesser palatine foramina

Pterygoid hamulus

Figure 12.1 The hard palate is formed by the palatine processes of the maxillae anteriorly and the horizontal processes of the palatine bones posteriorly. These bones meet in a cruciform suture system.

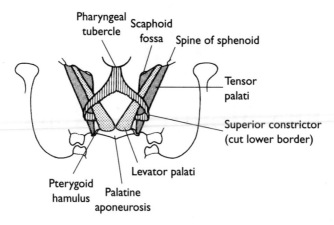

Figure 12.2 Diagrammatic representation of the muscles of the soft palate seen from behind. The tensor palati descends, outside the superior constrictor, from the scaphoid fossa and spine of the sphenoid bone to hook round the pterygoid hamulus and into the palatine aponeurosis. The levator palati passes over the top of the superior constrictor and descends into the top of the soft palate.

membrane towards the front of the hard palate is raised into ridges called **rugae**. There are also mucous glands and minor salivary glands in the palate. The rugae are important in speech and eating. They assist when eating by rubbing food into the surface of the tongue and contribute to the ability to taste things and judge texture.

A flat **palatine aponeurosis** attaches to the posterior edge of the hard palate. The muscles of the soft palate insert into this tough sheet. There are five muscles on each side of the soft palate. The soft palate is very mobile and moves and contracts in a complex manner when we speak and swallow. The **levator palati** and the **tensor palati** both arise from the base of the skull near the auditory tube. They can be seen on their way down to the palate in Figure 12.2. The levator passes over the top of the superior constrictor at its upper border (running through the pharyngobasilar fascia here) and spreads out on top of the aponeurosis to insert into it. It approaches its fellow on the other side at the midline. This muscle elevates the palate.

The tensor palati descends from the cranial base as a triangular sheet. It originates from the **scaphoid fossa** of the sphenoid bone in front (just between the roots of the two pterygoid plates) and from the **spine of the sphenoid** bone behind (just by the foramen spinosum). From these two bony points of origin it then converges inferiorly onto the pterygoid hamulus as a tendon. The tensor curls around this structure using it as a pulley. Its course is now more or less horizontal into the palatine aponeurosis. The tensor

palati acts to flatten the domed soft palate when it contracts.

The **palatoglossus** and **palatopharyngeus** muscles run from the aponeurosis and descend into the tongue and pharynx respectively (Fig. 12.3). Two slips of the palatopharyngeus embrace the lower end of levator palati on the top of the soft palate. The palatopharyngeus descends into the pharynx where it attaches on to the thyroid lamina. Palatoglossus arises from the undersurface of the aponeurosis and runs into the side of the tongue. During their descent these two muscles create two ridges of mucous membrane called the palatoglossal and palatopharyngeal arches. These are the so-called anterior and posterior **pillars of the fauces** respectively. The palatoglossal arch forms the posterior boundary of the cavity of the mouth. Between the two arches is a fossa which contains the palatine tonsil. The palatopharyngeus also acts as a constrictor muscle at the entrance to the oropharynx. The **musculus uvulae** is essentially an intrinsic muscle of the soft palate. It arises from the posterior edge of the hard palate in the midline and runs into a small tongue-like flap, called the **uvula**, which hangs from the posterior edge of the soft palate. This muscle raises a midline bulge in the upper surface of the soft palate during swallowing, which acts as a bung to help close off the nasopharynx from the mouth.

The nerve supply to the palate is best thought of with the pharynx in mind. Motor supply to both pharyngeal and palatine muscles is through the **vagoaccessory complex** in the **pharyngeal plexus**

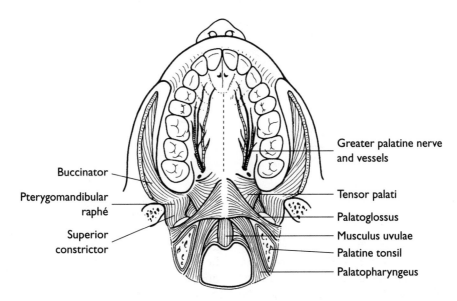

Figure 12.3 Palatopharyngeus and palatoglossus run down from the soft palate and form the folds of the anterior and posterior pillars of the fauces, between which the palatine tonsil lies.

and through the **laryngeal nerves** as well. There are two exceptions in the palate and pharynx. The tensor palati is supplied by a small nerve from the region of the otic ganglion, that is by the mandibular division of the trigeminal nerve (Viii). The stylopharyngeus is in intimate relationship with the glossopharyngeal nerve (the IXth cranial nerve) and is supplied by it. Sensory supply in the pharynx depends on the level. The roof of the nasopharynx and nose is supplied by the maxillary division of the trigeminal nerve (Vii). The palatine branches of this supply much of the palate, both hard and soft. The oropharynx, mucous membrane of the auditory tube, tonsil and a little of the soft palate is supplied by the glossopharyngeal nerve (IX). The laryngopharynx is supplied with sensation by the vagus nerve (the Xth cranial nerve).

The floor of the mouth

Two muscles run into the floor of the mouth from the skull base and another spans the mandible from side to side. Together they form a muscular bed for the tongue to rest on and provide a framework for two important salivary glands, the **submandibular** and **sublingual glands**. The posterior belly of the digastric arises as a fleshy belly from a groove on the inner side of the mastoid process (Fig. 12.4). The posterior belly tapers to a tendon which slides through a fibrous sling attached near the lesser cornu of the hyoid bone. A synovial sheath surrounds this intermediate tendon. The anterior belly of the digastric passes forwards on the undersurface of the mylohyoid muscle and inserts into the lower border of the mandible beneath the chin. It depresses the chin and opens the mouth when it acts with the lateral pterygoid muscle. It can also raise the hyoid bone when the teeth are clenched (as when swallowing, for example).

Note the relationship of the infrahyoid strap muscles to the mylohyoid and stylohyoid (Fig. 12.4). The stylohyoid muscle arises from the styloid process. It runs along the upper border of the digastric muscle. At the hyoid bone, the tendon of insertion splits and inserts into the greater cornu of the hyoid. The intermediate tendon of the digastric passes through the split in the stylohyoid tendon. The posterior belly of the digastric and the stylohyoid are derivatives of the second pharyngeal arch and are therefore supplied by the facial nerve (the VIIth cranial nerve).

The stylohyoid retracts and elevates the hyoid and is active during swallowing. The mylohyoid forms a sling or diaphragm across the floor of the mouth. The muscle arises on both sides from the inner aspect of the mandible. Here it raises an oblique ridge on the body of the mandible called the **mylohyoid line**. The

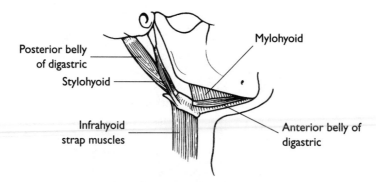

Figure 12.4 Stylohyoid splits at its insertion into the greater horn of the hyoid bone to pass either side of the intermediate tendon of the digastric muscle. The intermediate tendon can slide through a fibrous sling here.

mylohyoid inserts into the front of the body of the hyoid bone. It also meets in the midline at a raphé or seam which extends from the front of the hyoid bone to the mandibular symphysis anteriorly. Like the digastric and stylohyoid, the mylohyoid can also elevate the hyoid bone (Fig. 12.4). Its contraction thereby raises the whole floor of the mouth. The mylohyoid is supplied by a branch of the mandibular nerve that leaves the inferior alveolar nerve by the mandibular foramen at the posterior end of the mylohyoid line. This nerve is the motor supply for the mylohyoid and the anterior belly of the digastric. They are clearly therefore muscles derived from the first pharyngeal arch.

Look once again at the branches of the external carotid artery (Fig. 12.5). The facial artery at first lies deep to the digastric and stylohyoid muscles and on the surface of the superior constrictor lateral to the tonsillar fossa. The facial artery gives an important branch here, which pierces the superior constrictor to reach the tonsillar bed. It then passes up and over the top of the digastric and stylohyoid, and down to the free posterior edge of the mylohyoid. Here it is in contact with the submandibular salivary gland. At this point it lies against the inner aspect of the body of the mandible. From here it curls round the lower border of the mandible and up into the face.

The submandibular salivary gland is sandwiched between the muscles of the floor of the mouth. Part of it is squeezed out on to the external surface of the mylohyoid underneath the floor of the mouth. This is where the facial artery grooves the gland and is

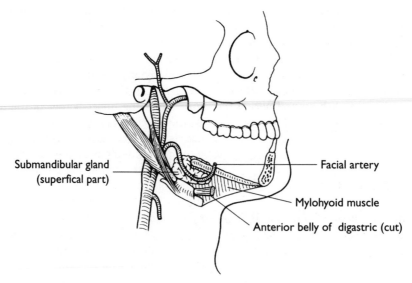

Figure 12.5 The facial artery arises deep to the digastric and stylohyoid muscles. It hooks over the top of them and passes over, or through, the submandibular gland near the free posterior border of the mylohyoid muscle. From here it curls beneath the lower border of the mandible, just anterior to the insertion of masseter, and runs up into the face.

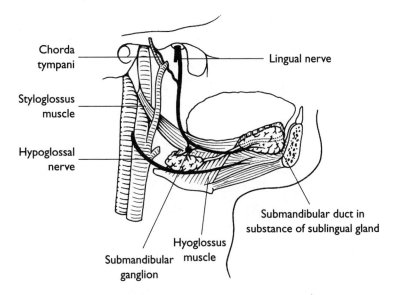

Chorda tympani

Lingual nerve

Styloglossus muscle

Hypoglossal nerve

Submandibular duct in substance of sublingual gland

Hyoglossus muscle

Submandibular ganglion

Figure 12.6 The chorda tympani joins the lingual nerve high in the infratemporal fossa. Parasympathetic nerve fibres travelling in the chorda tympani synapse in the submandibular ganglion suspended below the lingual nerve. The hypoglossal nerve passes lateral to both internal and external carotid arteries and then below the submandibular gland lateral to the hyoglossus muscle.

sometimes even found in the substance of the gland here (Fig. 12.5). Removal of the digastric, stylohyoid and mylohyoid muscles together with the facial artery and superficial part of the submandibular gland reveals another group of muscles within the floor of the mouth, as well as the main body and duct of the submandibular gland and two more nerves (Fig. 12.6).

The muscles that are now seen in this deep plane act on the tongue. They are the **hyoglossus** and the **styloglossus**. The hyoglossus is square in its lateral outline and arises from the sides of the hyoid, passing up to insert into the tongue. It pulls the tongue down into the mouth. The styloglossus passes from the styloid process, between the external and internal carotid arteries, to enter the back of the tongue. All the muscles of the tongue except palatoglossus are supplied by the **hypoglossal nerve.**

The submandibular and sublingual salivary glands

The bulk of the submandibular salivary gland is visible in Figures 12.5 and 12.6, as is also the smaller sublingual gland (Fig. 12.6). The submandibular gland is a mixed salivary gland, that is to say it contains both serous and mucous-secreting acini. The sublingual gland contains only mucous-secreting acini. The submandibular gland consists of a deep and superficial part. It is the deep part that is found on the surface of the hyoglossus and, although difficult to conceive, it is the superficial part that lies on the inferior surface of the mylohyoid, in reality in the neck. The lingual nerve lies above the submandibular gland and the hypoglossal nerve (the XIIth cranial nerve) below it. The submandibular duct leaves the deep part of the gland and opens at a small papilla in the floor of the mouth near the midline at the front under the tongue. It lies just to the side of the **lingual frenulum** that ties the tip of the tongue to the mucous membrane of the floor of the mouth. If you look into your own mouth here and think of chewing into a lemon, for example, this will become clear to you.

The lingual nerve hooks underneath the submandibular duct before ascending medial to it and up into the tongue (Fig. 12.7). Stones are occasionally formed in the submandibular gland and can block the duct. They can be felt in the floor of the mouth and are usually removed by opening the duct through the mucous membrane in the floor of the mouth.

The sublingual gland lies close to the lingual nerve just deep to the mucous membrane of the floor of the mouth under the tongue. It is drained by several small ducts, some entering the submandibular duct and others opening directly into the floor of the mouth.

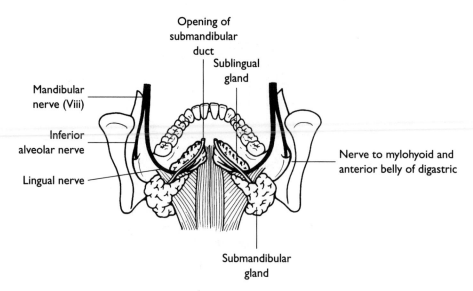

Opening of
submandibular
duct

Sublingual
gland

Mandibular
nerve (Viii)

Inferior
alveolar nerve

Lingual nerve

Nerve to mylohyoid and
anterior belly of digastric

Submandibular
gland

Figure 12.7 The lingual nerve comes to lie on the bone of the mandible close to the roots of the lower third molar tooth. It then passes medially and hooks beneath the submandibular duct before rising up into the substance of the tongue.

The hypoglossal nerve

The lingual branch of the mandibular division of the trigeminal nerve (Viii) and the hypoglossal nerve (the XIIth cranial nerve) both have important relations in the floor of the mouth. The hypoglossal nerve is the motor nerve to all the muscles of the tongue except palatoglossus. It leaves the skull through the anterior condylar foramen. To gain the interval between the internal carotid artery and internal jugular vein, the nerve has to swing outwards very markedly. At the level of the hyoid bone the hypoglossal nerve loops around the external carotid artery at the point at which the occipital branch and the lingual branch of the external carotid arise. In this way it comes to run closely with the lingual artery just below the lower border of the digastric muscle. The hypoglossal nerve is quite superficial in this part of its course. From this position it passes on to the outer aspect of the hyoglossus muscle where it breaks up into twigs which supply all the tongue musculature. The lingual artery by contrast passes *deep* to hyoglossus at its posterior border. For the sake of completion, note again that during part of its course the hypoglossal nerve carries some fibres from cervical segment C1 which 'hitch-hike' along it to the thyrohyoid and geniohyoid muscles.

The lingual nerve

The lingual nerve is a particularly important branch of the mandibular division of the Vth cranial nerve (Viii). It lies first on the lateral surface of the medial pterygoid muscle and then against the mandible next to the roots of the last molar tooth (Fig. 12.7). From here it enters the floor of the mouth with the styloglossus muscle. It is the general sensory nerve to the anterior two-thirds of the tongue and floor of the mouth. The lingual nerve also supplies general sensation to the gingivae on the lingual aspect of the teeth and alveolar bone of the mandible. However, the lingual nerve also has two other important functions. It carries special taste sensation from the anterior two-thirds of the tongue and parasympathetic neurons to the submandibular and sublingual glands. Look for a moment at the way in which this occurs (Fig. 12.6). The chorda tympani branch of the facial nerve (the VIIth cranial nerve) has already been mentioned in our study of the ear and infratemporal fossa.

Special taste fibres leave the tongue in the lingual nerve and pass back through the chorda tympani to join the VIIth nerve in the middle ear cavity. Parasympathetic preganglionic neurons destined for the submandibular and sublingual glands leave the brain in the VIIth cranial nerve and also pass into

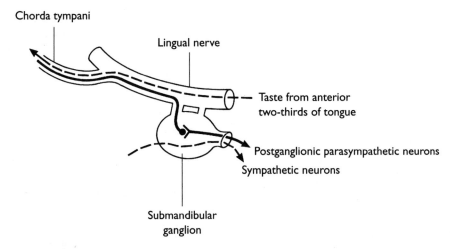

Figure 12.8 Postganglionic parasympathetic nerve fibres pass from the submandibular ganglion to innervate the submandibular and sublingual salivary glands as well as other minor salivary glands. Sympathetic nerve fibres pass through the ganglion without synapsing.

the chorda tympani. They travel down in it and join the lingual nerve but then pass to their ganglion, the **submandibular ganglion**, which hangs from the lingual nerve. This ganglion lies between the sub-mandibular gland and the hyoglossus (Figs 12.6 and 12.8). Within the ganglion preganglionic fibres synapse and then postganglionic parasympathetic neurons go on to the salivary glands and mucous glands of the floor of the mouth. Sympathetic fibres pass directly through the ganglion without synapse and are also involved in secretomotor activity of salivary and mucous glands, as well as being vaso-constrictor in function.

The genioglossus and geniohyoid muscles

The hyoglossus, both submandibular and sublingual salivary glands, and the two nerves may now be removed in order to see the deep muscles (Fig. 12.9). One muscle moves the hyoid bone and the other the tongue. Both arise from little bony spines, called **genial spines**, on the inner aspect of the mandible near the midline. The geniohyoid arises from the inside of the mandible at the front near the midline and passes back to insert into the body of the hyoid bone. Look at Figure 12.9 and note that the muscle is positioned to pull the hyoid upwards and forwards. The for-ward movement is opposed by the stylohyoid and

the upward movement by the infrahyoid strap muscles. The geniohyoid is supplied by those fibres from cervical segment C1 that have 'hitch-hiked' along the hypoglossal nerve.

The genioglossus forms a great deal of the bulk of the tongue. It also arises from the inside of the mandible near the midline. From here it spreads widely to insert into the whole length of the undersurface of the tongue. Like all the tongue muscles, genioglossus is supplied by the hypoglossal nerve (XII).

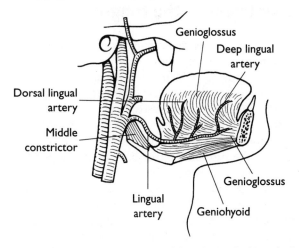

Figure 12.9 When hyoglossus and the submandibular and sub-lingual glands are removed, the genioglossus and geniohyoid muscles become visible. The lingual artery can now be seen its entirety since it runs deep to hyoglossus, on the surface of genioglossus. It gives dorsal branches to the back of the tongue and deep branches which run beneath the front and tip of the tongue.

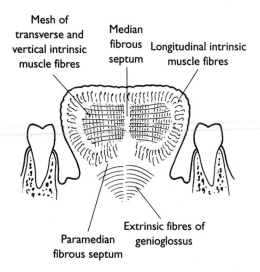

Mesh of transverse and vertical intrinsic muscle fibres

Median fibrous septum

Longitudinal intrinsic muscle fibres

Paramedian fibrous septum

Extrinsic fibres of genioglossus

Figure 12.10   The intrinsic muscles of the tongue alter the shape of the tongue. They form a weave of muscle fibres arranged around fibrous septa that run anteroposteriorly through the dorsum of the tongue. (After Tonge CH and Luke DA (1981) The tongue. *Dental Update* **8**: 79–87.)

The lingual artery can now be seen clearly. Having passed deep to hyoglossus, it gives branches into the tongue as it courses on the surface of the genioglossus.

The intrinsic muscles and mucous membrane of the tongue

The tongue has **extrinsic muscles** which take origin from bone and which move it as a whole, as well as **intrinsic muscles** which alter its shape. We have already studied the extrinsic muscles of the tongue: the **styloglossus, palatoglossus, hyoglossus** and **genioglossus**. The intrinsic muscles of the tongue form a weave of longitudinal, transverse and vertical muscle fibres in the substance of the body of the tongue (Fig. 12.10). Fibrous septa pass between these muscle fibres and form a flexible framework for the dorsum and tip of the tongue. All of these extrinsic and intrinsic muscles except palatoglossus are supplied by the hypoglossal nerve (XII). Lesions of the hypoglossal nerve can be detected by asking patients to stick their tongue out. The tongue swings over to the side of the lesion if there is hypoglossal nerve damage.

The structure and innervation of the tongue reflects its developmental history. The division between the anterior two-thirds and posterior one-third is marked on the dorsum of the tongue by a faint 'V-shaped' line called the **sulcus terminalis** (Fig. 12.11). In the midline, at the apex of the 'V', there is a shallow pit called the **foramen caecum** which represents the origin of the thyroid gland in the floor of the primitive pharynx. The mucous membrane of the surface of the tongue is firmly adherent to its surface and is referred to as **gustatory epithelium**. Beneath the tip of the tongue there is a median fold of mucous membrane, called the **frenulum**. This separates the two submandibular duct orifices. Posteriorly, there is a midline fold of mucous membrane which passes back to the epiglottis. This **median glossoepiglottic fold** separates the two **valleculae**.

The gustatory mucous membrane of the anterior two-thirds of the tongue contains four types of papillae. The **circumvallate papillae** are quite large and notable, and are arranged along the sulcus terminalis. Each is about 2 mm in diameter. On the anterior one-third of the tongue the rounded **fungiform papillae** appear red because they are not keratinized. The **filiform papillae** are rougher and are keratinized. The **foliate papillae** have deep folds between them on the side of the tongue near the sulcus terminalis. The posterior one-third of the tongue is roughened by collections of lymphoid tissue in the mucous membrane.

The lingual artery

The lingual artery is a major branch of the external carotid. It arises close to the hyoid bone and then forms a characteristic loop as it passes forwards on to the middle constrictor. We mentioned earlier that it runs into the tongue by travelling deep to the hyoglossus muscle (Fig. 12.9). As it does this it lies on the outer surface of the genioglossus. The main branches of the lingual artery are the **dorsal lingual arteries**, which run up to supply the dorsum of the tongue, and the **deep lingual arteries**, which continue to the tip and undersurface. The dorsal branches of the lingual artery also contribute to the supply of the palatine tonsil. The prominent blue veins visible on the undersurface of the tip of the tongue are branches of the deep lingual veins which accompany the arteries of the same name.

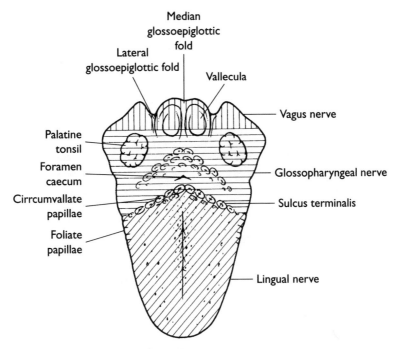

Median
glossoepiglottic
fold

Lateral
glossoepiglottic fold

Vallecula

Vagus nerve

Palatine
tonsil

Foramen
caecum

Cirrcumvallate
papillae

Foliate
papillae

Glossopharyngeal nerve

Sulcus terminalis

Lingual nerve

Figure 12.11 The sulcus terminalis divides the tongue into anterior two-thirds and posterior one-third. These are supplied with general sensation by the lingual nerve and the glossopharyngeal nerve respectively. The vagus supplies the most posterior part of the tongue adjacent to the epiglottis. Taste fibres from the anterior two-thirds run in the chorda tympani and from the posterior one-third in the glossopharyngeal nerve.

Innervation of the tongue

General sensation from the anterior two-thirds of the tongue is conveyed in the lingual nerve (Fig. 12.11). General sensation from the posterior one-third of the tongue is conveyed in the glossopharyngeal nerve (the XIIth cranial nerve). Taste from the anterior two-thirds of the tongue is conveyed in the chorda tympani via the lingual nerve to the facial nerve in the petrous temporal bone. Taste fibres from the posterior one-third of the tongue travel in the glossopharyngeal nerve (the IXth cranial nerve). A small part of the back of the tongue adjacent to the epiglottis and piriform fossae receives general sensory fibres that run in the vagus nerve (the Xth cranial nerve).

The face

The superficial musculature of the face surrounds the ear, nose, orbit and mouth. As a group these muscles are known as the **muscles of facial**

expression. The facial muscles form sphincters and dilators around each of these orifices. There is little virtue in learning the names of every facial muscle but one or two are important and the principles of what they all do is important. All of the muscles of facial expression are supplied by the facial nerve (the VIIth cranial nerve). We have followed the path of this nerve into the internal acoustic meatus and through the petrous temporal bone and middle ear. We have seen it appear in the infratemporal fossa as it emerges through the stylomastoid foramen. The final pathway of this nerve can now be studied in detail, together with details of the facial artery in the face.

The most important muscles of the face are labelled in Figure 12.12. Notice first the muscle around the eye, the **orbicularis oculi**. Its fibres form a sphincter around the eye. We studied its palpebral and orbital parts with the structures of the orbit. A large muscle called the **frontalis** lies above the eyes in the scalp. The frontalis is attached to the epicranial aponeurosis superiorly. At the back of the vault there is another muscle called the

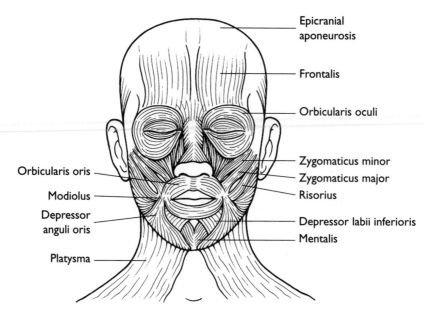

Epicranial
aponeurosis

Frontalis

Orbicularis oculi

Zygomaticus minor

Zygomaticus major

Risorius

Depressor labii inferioris

Mentalis

Orbicularis oris

Modiolus

Depressor
anguli oris

Platysma

Figure 12.12 The muscles of facial expression (and the buccinator muscle) are all supplied by the the facial, VIIth, cranial nerve.

occipitalis, which attaches to the epicranial aponeurosis anteriorly. The whole structure, occipitalis, epicranial aponeurosis and frontalis, is called the **occipitofrontalis**.

The mouth is also surrounded by a large circular sphincter muscle. This is called the **orbicularis oris**. Orbicularis oris has no bony origin. Around it, arranged in a radial manner, are muscles that raise the upper lip, raise or depress the corner of the mouth, and depress the lower lip. Their names describe their actions but need not be learned. A few of their names appear in Figure 12.12.

At this point it is important not to forget the **buccinator muscle**, which lies on a deeper plane in the side of the cheek. This is also, strictly speaking, a muscle of facial expression and is supplied by the facial nerve.

There is, of course, no strong sphincter muscle around the nose, since this would be a distinct disadvantage, but there are some small muscles that dilatate the nostrils and act as important accessory muscles of respiration (more so in other animals though). Similarly, small muscles around the ear, which some of us can use, are far more important in other animals than in humans. Finally, we should remember the platysma muscle in the neck, which is also a muscle of facial expression and is supplied by the facial nerve.

The facial artery in the face

The **facial artery** leaves the external carotid artery near the lingual artery and reaches the border of the mandible just anterior to the masseter muscle. From here it runs a 'tortuous' or twisting course past the angle of the mouth and side of the nose (Fig. 12.13). This allows for movements of the face and jaws. When the jaw is opened widely, as when yawning for example, the facial artery is stretched such that its course is straighter. At the side of the nose the facial artery is renamed the **angular artery**. It passes to the medial angle of the eye and anastomoses with orbital vessels here. Some terminal branches also continue into the scalp to anastomose there. It gives **labial branches** to the lips, and branches to the external nose also. It also gives a branch that passes obliquely back across the cheek. This anastomoses with the **transverse facial branch** of the **superficial temporal artery**.

The **facial vein** accompanies the artery. Both the vein and the artery pass deep to the **zygomaticus major** in the cheek but only the artery passes deep to the **zygomaticus minor** on its way to the medial angle of the eye. The vein remains more superficial here. The facial vein communicates with the orbital veins and intracranial venous sinuses. The vein joins the anterior branch of the retromandibular vein to form the common facial vein which drains into the internal jugular vein.

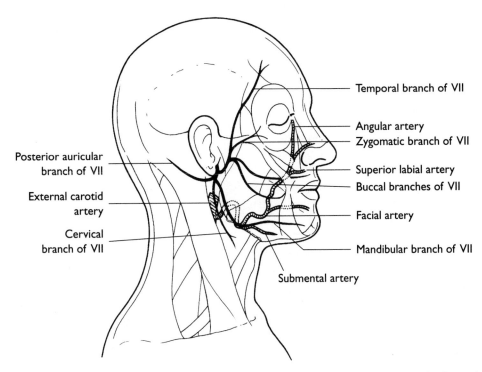

Figure 12.13 The facial artery runs deep to both zygomaticus major and minor. It gives branches to the lips and external nose before becoming the angular artery. The facial nerve (VII) emerges from the parotid gland from where it gives motor branches to each of the muscles of facial expression (and to the stylohyoid and posterior belly of the digastric muscle).

The facial nerve in the face

The facial nerve is also found superficially in the face (Fig. 12.13). It is entirely motor and supplies all the muscles of facial expression we have described in this area, including buccinator. It passes through the superficial substance of the parotid gland, dividing into its terminal branches within the gland. The nerve lies superficial to the retromandibular vein and external carotid artery and the terminal branches of this artery in the gland. The terminal branches of the facial nerve pass upwards to the temporal region (**temporal branches**), across the zygomatic arch (**zygomatic branches**), across the cheek (**buccal branches**), along the mandible (**mandibular branches**) and into the neck (**cervical branches**). The cervical branch innervates the platysma muscle. A small **posterior auricular** branch passes back to supply the posterior belly of the digastric and the stylohyoid muscles.

Sensory supply to the skin of the face and forehead is through cutaneous branches of the three divisions of the trigeminal nerve. The dermatomes are shown in Figure 12.14. Light touch, pressure, temperature and pain are all conveyed to the trigeminal nuclei in the brain via the three divisions of the trigeminal nerve. Each of these sensations can be tested clinically and mapped out on the face in the distributions of each division of the nerve to its dermatome.

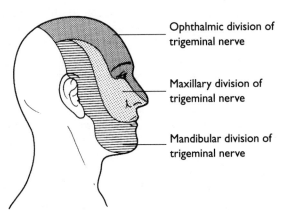

Figure 12.14 The sensory nerve supply to the face and much of the scalp is through the three divisions of the trigeminal, Vth, nerve.

Applied anatomy of the mouth and face

Swallowing, or **deglutition,** is a vitally important process that occurs many times a day and is controlled by reflexes that involve the IXth, Xth and XIth cranial nerves in the brain stem. The two things fundamental to the swallowing mechanism are that food is prevented from entering the nose and the airway. Choking and food passing up into the nose, for example, are both symptoms of **bulbar palsy,** which is a degeneration of the nuclei of cranial nerves IX and X. The **first stage** of swallowing is voluntary and involves movements of the tongue in the mouth. The tongue is raised and pressed against the roof of the mouth and the bolus of food is moved back towards the oropharynx. As this happens the teeth come together to stabilize the mandible so that many muscles can act from it during the second and third stages of swallowing. As soon as food comes into contact with the back of the tongue and the part of the oropharynx innervated by the glossopharyngeal nerve (the IXth cranial nerve), the **second stage** of swallowing begins. This is involuntary and after the beginning of this stage one cannot suddenly decide to stop swallowing. During the second stage of swallowing the soft palate is raised and tensed against the posterior wall of the pharynx to prevent food entering the nose. The pharynx also constricts here at the **pharyngeal isthmus** as part of this mechanism. The bolus of food is passed back into the oropharynx by the tongue and contractions of the pharyngeal constrictor muscles move it down through the oropharynx towards the laryngopharynx. As this occurs there is first an anterior movement of the hyoid bone and then a raising of the hyoid bone in the neck. This is quickly followed by elevation of the larynx (by the equivalent of two cervical vertebral segments). The larynx is therefore pulled upwards and forwards to the back of the base of the tongue. The aryepiglottic muscles have a very important sphincteric action at this time around the laryngeal inlet. There are also other muscle fibres in the wall of the inlet that contribute to this sphincteric tightening of the laryngeal inlet. When contracted they also help to guide food and drink either side of the laryngeal inlet. The **third stage** of swallowing involves the inferior constrictor muscle squeezing the bolus of food out of the laryngopharynx

through the **cricopharyngeal sphincter** and into the oesophagus.

Cleft palate and cleft lip are congenital abnormalities that arise through incomplete fusion of the maxillary

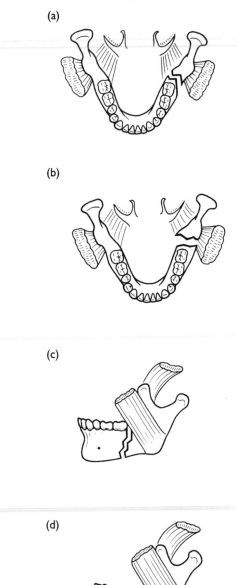

Figure 12.15   In (a) the pull of the left lateral pterygoid muscle draws the fractured portions of the mandible together. In (b) it pulls them apart such that the fracture is said to be unfavourable. In (c) the masseter and temporalis muscles again draw the fractured mandible together, whereas in (d) they act to separate the fracture, which is oriented unfavourably. (After Killey HC (1974) *Fractures of the Mandible.* Bristol: J. Wright and Sons.)

processes of the mandibular arch during development. Clefts are either unilateral or bilateral. They may result simply from failure of fusion of the embryonic process, for whatever reason. One cause may be that the maxillary processes are held apart by the developing tongue which remains high if the fetus fails to unflex. The tongue is unable to drop into the developing mouth in these circumstances. Clefts are best described and classified with reference to the structures they affect. They may involve the lip only (hare lip). They may involve the lip and alveolar process of the maxilla, or even extend into the hard and soft palate as well. Clefts of the palate may be as minor as bifid uvula, which is of little consequence. Soon after birth cleft lips are repaired. Cleft palates are repaired a bit later, initially by freeing the mucosa from the bone of the hard palate on each side and bringing them together in the midline. Attempts at bony repair are carried out later in childhood.

Fractures of the mandible are common. Some fractures are left to remodel without treatment, such as fractures to the mandibular condyles. These typically follow a blow to the chin. Other fractures are more serious and can occur in many places along the body or at the chin, or across the ascending ramus. Fractures such as these require fixation. The direction of the fracture line determines whether or not the muscles of mastication hold the broken ends of the bone in place. Unfavourable fractures tend to pull apart. Favourable fractures are held together by the contraction of the masticatory muscles (Fig. 12.15).

The facial nerve can be tested by asking patients to screw up their eyes and show their teeth. Inability to do this on one or other side of the face indicates a **facial nerve palsy** (or **Bell's palsy**). Commonly this follows inflammation of the facial nerve in the facial canal in the petrous temporal bone.

An upper motor neuron lesion affecting the facial nerve, such as a stroke, presents differently. Since fibres from the right and left sides of the brain both innervate the muscles above the level of the eye, the orbicularis oculi remains unaffected in upper motor neuron lesions on one side of the brain. However, the lower facial muscles receive fibres from only one side of the brain and are therefore unable to perform voluntary movements in upper motor neuron lesions of the same side of the brain, as they are in Bell's palsy. So patients suffering damage to the VIIth cranial nerve due to a stroke can still voluntarily move the muscles around the eye and forehead, unlike those with a Bell's facial palsy who cannot.

It is important to be able to recognize the dermatomes of the trigeminal nerve for other reasons. The Herpes zoster virus can survive in the satellite cells surrounding the trigeminal ganglion for years. In older people or in those who are 'run down' or otherwise susceptible, it can travel down one or other division of the Vth cranial nerve and present as a vesicular rash in the exact distribution of the dermatome involved. A good knowledge of dermatomes in the head and neck, as well as in the trunk, allows a precise and instant diagnosis of this kind of lesion.

chapter

13

Summary and Revision of the Infratemporal Fossa, Nose, Mouth and Face

First, read through the following summaries of all the cranial nerves that we have described in the infratemporal fossa, nose and mouth. Use Figure 13.1 to help you. Make sure you understand how to test each of them and that you are clear about their course through these different regions. Some of the multiple choice questions that follow require a knowledge of facts given in these summaries. So that you bring together what you have learned about the infratemporal fossa, the nose, the mouth and the face, go through the multiple choice questions at the end of this chapter. For each **stem**, any one of the five answers (A)–(E) may be either correct or incorrect. You may choose to do them all on one occasion or you may choose to do alternate questions at your first attempt and then the others on a subsequent occasion. Many of these questions are intentionally quite searching. A score of around 50% correct would be quite reasonable at your first attempt. We expect you to have to refer back to the text to improve your score on subsequent attempts. In so doing you will improve your understanding of head and neck anatomy.

Summary of cranial nerves Vii, Viii, VII and XII

Cranial nerve Vii

We described the first division, the ophthalmic division, of the trigeminal nerve together with the nerves associated with the orbit. The second, or maxillary, division also runs in the lateral wall of the cavernous sinus. It is the sensory nerve to the midface, nasal cavity and palate as well as to the lower eyelid and associated

conjunctiva. Its branches in the infratemporal fossa include the infraorbital, greater palatine and nasopalatine branches. These run respectively forwards into the cheek, downwards into the hard and soft palate, and medially into the nose and roof of the nasopharynx. Alveolar branches are also given off in the infratemporal fossa. These pass inferiorly to the maxillary teeth and maxillary antrum. The maxillary division is entirely sensory, but each of its branches picks up postganglionic parasympathetic secretomotor fibres from the greater superficial petrosal branch of the facial nerve that have synapsed in the pterygopalatine ganglion. These travel with its branches to glands in the nasal mucosa and on the palate. The maxillary nerve can be tested through response to touch, pressure, pain (such as a pinprick) and temperature over its distribution on the cheek, temple, upper lip and lower eyelid.

Cranial nerve Viii

The mandibular division of the trigeminal nerve passes through the foramen ovale and into the roof of the infratemporal fossa. Its anterior division gives motor branches to all the muscles of mastication and to the tensor tympani and tensor palati muscles. It gives one sensory branch to the inside of the cheek called the long buccal branch and another small spinosus branch which runs up with the middle meningeal artery. This supplies dura in the middle cranial fossa and also helps supply the mucous membrane of the mastoid air cells. The posterior division of the mandibular branch divides into the auriculotemporal nerve, inferior alveolar nerve, the lingual nerve and a small motor branch to the mylohyoid and anterior belly of the digastric muscle. The auriculotemporal nerve passes laterally, splitting to pass either side of the middle meningeal artery. It supplies the skin of the temple, scalp and front of the auricle here and the anterior portion of the external auditory meatus. It also picks up postganglionic parasympathetic fibres from the lesser superficial petrosal branch of the glossopharyngeal nerve that have

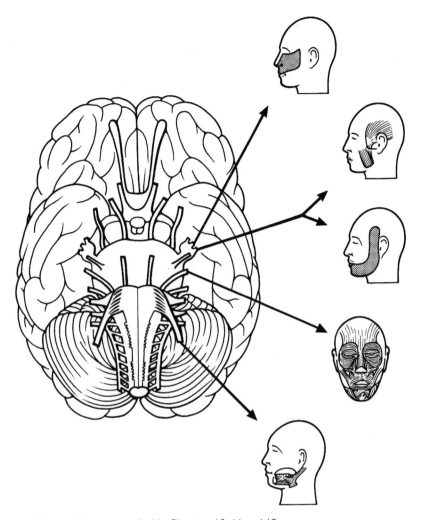

Figure 13.1 Summary of the cranial nerves studied in Chapters 10, 11 and 12.

synapsed in the otic ganglion, and carries them to the parotid gland. The inferior alveolar nerve supplies the pulp cavities of the teeth with sensation and then emerges through the mental foramen as the mental nerve to supply the skin and mucous membrane of the lower lip and the skin over the chin. The lingual nerve runs over the lateral surface of the medial pterygoid muscle and then runs on to the bone of the mandible where it lies just beneath the third molar tooth roots. It then passes medially across the floor of the mouth, hooking underneath the submandibular duct, before it runs up into the substance of the tongue. It carries general sensation to the anterior two-thirds of the tongue. The lingual nerve is also joined, high in the infratemporal fossa, by the chorda tympani branch of the facial nerve. We last described this branch as it left the middle ear via the petrotympanic fissure. The chorda tympani carries preganglionic parasympathetic nerve fibres to the submandibular ganglion. These relay here, and postganglionic fibres continue as secretomotor nerves to the submandibular and sublingual

salivary glands. Taste sensation from the anterior two-thirds of the tongue joins the chorda tympani and runs back to the facial nerve in the middle ear. The mandibular nerve can be tested by asking a subject to bite their teeth together on both sides and to protrude the lower jaw. The sensory component of the nerve can be tested in the same way as the maxillary division over the dermatome of this nerve in the lower face.

Cranial nerve VII
The facial nerve leaves the skull through the stylomastoid foramen. It then enters the parotid gland and runs forwards through the substance of the gland superficially. At the margins of the gland it emerges as temporal, zygomatic, buccal, marginal mandibular and cervical branches. These are all motor nerves to the muscles of facial expression. The facial nerve can be tested by asking a subject to blink, screw their eyes up, show their teeth and/or whistle.

Cranial nerve XII

The hypoglossal nerve in the neck lies quite superficially, close to the lingual artery by the side of the hyoid bone. It then passes forwards and runs over the lateral aspect of the hyoglossus muscle in the floor of the mouth. Branches of the hypoglossal nerve run to each of the intrinsic and extrinsic muscles of the tongue (except palatoglossus). The nerve can be tested by asking a subject to stick their tongue out. The tongue deviates to the side of the lesion when the hypoglossal nerve is ineffective.

Multiple Choice Questions on the Infratemporal Fossa, Nose, Mouth and Face

I. The pterygopalatine fossa communicates with:
(A) the orbit through the inferior orbital fissure
(B) the nose through the sphenopalatine foramen
(C) the middle cranial fossa through the foramen rotundum
(D) the posterior cranial fossa through the pterygoid canal
(E) the middle cranial fossa through the foramen spinosum

A____ B____ C____ D____ E____

2. The trigeminal ganglion:
(A) lies in a depression on the petrous temporal bone
(B) has the internal carotid artery lying lateral to it
(C) contains the cell bodies of the sensory fibres of the Vth cranial nerve
(D) contains parasympathetic synapses
(E) lies entirely in the extradural space

A____ B____ C____ D____ E____

3. The maxillary nerve:
(A) is medial to the internal carotid artery in the cavernous sinus
(B) enters the orbit through the superior orbital fissure
(C) supplies sensation to the mucous membrane of the maxillary air sinus
(D) supplies sensation to the lower lip
(E) supplies sensation to the lower eyelid

A____ B____ C____ D____ E____

4. The trigeminal nerve:
(A) has a large sensory and a small motor root
(B) has three autonomic ganglia associated with its terminal branches
(C) carries taste fibres from the posterior one-third of the tongue
(D) has a mandibular division, which leaves the skull through the foramen rotundum
(E) has a maxillary division which is both sensory and motor

A____ B____ C____ D____ E____

5. The pterygopalatine ganglion:
(A) receives preganglionic parasympathetic secretomotor fibres from the greater superficial petrosal nerve
(B) receives preganglionic sympathetic fibres
(C) lies medial to the sphenopalatine foramen
(D) contains the nerve cell bodies of fibres destined to supply the lacrimal gland
(E) relays postganglionic parasympathetic secretomotor fibres to the parotid gland

A____ B____ C____ D____ E____

6. The lateral pterygoid muscle:
(A) elevates the mandible
(B) inserts into the coronoid process of the mandible
(C) has an insertion which, in part, is into the intra-articular disc of the temporomandibular joint
(D) is active while opening the mouth and protruding the mandible
(E) is supplied by the mandibular nerve (Vi)

A____ B____ C____ D____ E____

7. The temporomandibular joint:
(A) has a condyle covered with hyaline cartilage
(B) allows simple hinge movements in the lower joint compartment
(C) is formed between the zygomatic bone and the condyle of the mandible
(D) is an example of a secondary cartilaginous joint
(E) allows forward translation of the mandibular condyle

A____ B____ C____ D____ E____

8. The masseter muscle:
(A) takes origin from the lateral aspect of the lateral pterygoid plate
(B) has the parotid duct running through its substance
(C) has the facial artery close to its lower anterior border
(D) has part of the parotid gland lying on its lateral surface
(E) is supplied by the facial nerve (VII)

A____ B____ C____ D____ E____

9. The parotid gland:
(A) contains the facial nerve (VII) within its substance
(B) is encapsulated by deep cervical fascia
(C) is innervated by the hypoglossal nerve (XII) with secretomotor fibres
(D) has a duct that opens opposite the neck of the upper canine tooth
(E) has the internal carotid artery within its substance

A____ B____ C____ D____ E____

10. The maxillary sinus:
(A) drains via its ostium into the inferior meatus
(B) has the infraorbital nerve running in its bony roof
(C) has alveolar nerves destined for the teeth in its walls
(D) is well developed at birth
(E) has its opening at the same level as the floor of the sinus

A____ B____ C____ D____ E____

11. The following are found in the middle meatus of the lateral wall of the nose:
(A) the opening of the sphenoidal air sinus
(B) the opening of the maxillary air sinus
(C) the bulla ethmoidalis
(D) the opening of the frontal air sinus
(E) the opening of the nasolacrimal duct

A____ B____ C____ D____ E____

12. The palatine bone:
(A) has a horizontal part that forms the whole of the hard palate
(B) has a vertical part that sutures with the maxilla
(C) completely encircles the sphenopalatine foramen
(D) has a part called the pterygoid hamulus at the back of the hard palate
(E) can be seen from the side of a skull in the depths of the pterygopalatine fossa

A____ B____ C____ D____ E____

13. Branches of the maxillary division of the trigeminal nerve include:
(A) the mental nerve
(B) the infraorbital nerve
(C) the supraorbital nerve
(D) the zygomaticofacial nerve
(E) the anterior ethmoidal nerve

A____ B____ C____ D____ E____

14. The lingual nerve:
(A) is a branch of the maxillary division of the trigeminal nerve (Vii)
(B) carries parasympathetic fibres for the submandibular gland
(C) carries taste fibres from the anterior two-thirds of the tongue
(D) transmits general sensation from the anterior two-thirds of the tongue
(E) is joined by the chorda tympani

A____ B____ C____ D____ E____

15. The submandibular gland:
(A) is in direct relationship with part of the hyoglossus muscle
(B) has a duct under which the lingual nerve passes
(C) is related to the hypoglossal nerve
(D) receives secretomotor fibres from the facial nerve (VII)
(E) receives sympathetic nerve fibres

A____ B____ C____ D____ E____

16. The digastric muscle:
(A) has a posterior belly that arises deep to the mastoid process
(B) can depress the mandible
(C) can elevate the hyoid bone
(D) receives a nerve supply from both facial (VII) and mandibular (Vi) nerves
(E) is closely related to the occipital and posterior auricular branches of the external carotid artery

A____ B____ C____ D____ E____

17. The buccinator muscle:
(A) is the lowermost part of the superior constrictor muscle
(B) is supplied by the facial nerve (VII)
(C) is pierced by the parotid duct
(D) takes part in the formation of the modiolus
(E) assists in opening the mouth

A____ B____ C____ D____ E____

18. Structures found in the interval between the mylohyoid and hyoglossus include:
(A) the lingual artery
(B) the submandibular duct
(C) the lingual nerve
(D) the glossopharyngeal nerve
(E) the anterior belly of digastric

A____ B____ C____ D____ E____

19. The tongue:
(A) has taste fibres from its anterior two-thirds that travel to the facial nerve (VII)
(B) has extrinsic and intrinsic muscles that are supplied by the lingual nerve
(C) is depressed in the mouth by the action of the hyoglossus
(D) is directly attached to the mandible along the mylohyoid line
(E) receives general sensation to its posterior one-third via the glossopharyngeal nerve (IX)

A____ B____ C____ D____ E____

20. The glossopharyngeal nerve:
(A) is motor to the palatoglossus
(B) is motor to the posterior belly of the digastric muscle
(C) gives a branch to the carotid body and carotid sinus
(D) carries taste fibres from the posterior one-third of the tongue
(E) conducts ordinary sensation from the posterior one-third of the tongue

A____ B____ C____ D____ E____

21. Postganglionic fibres from the submandibular ganglion supply:
(A) the hyoglossus muscle
(B) taste buds on the tongue
(C) the facial artery (vasoconstrictor)
(D) sweat glands in the skin of the chin
(E) the sublingual salivary glands

A____ B____ C____ D____ E____

22. The sublingual gland:
(A) is covered with a capsule of investing deep cervical fascia
(B) receives secretomotor fibres from the submandibular ganglion
(C) has only mucus-secreting acini
(D) opens via a single duct just lateral to the lingual frenulum
(E) has a part which lies superficially in the neck

A____ B____ C____ D____ E____

23. The facial artery:
(A) gives branches that supply the palatine tonsil
(B) runs through the parotid gland for part of its course
(C) can be felt pulsing at the lower anterior border of the masseter muscle
(D) gives branches to both upper and lower lips
(E) anastomoses with the ophthalmic artery, a branch of the internal carotid artery, at the medial angle of the eye

A____ B____ C____ D____ E____

24. Concerning the muscles of facial expression:
(A) the orbicularis oris has no bony attachments
(B) they are all supplied by the facial nerve (VII)
(C) the orbicularis oculi has a dual motor nerve supply
(D) patients with a facial nerve palsy (Bell's palsy) are unable to blink
(E) patients with an upper motor neuron lesion of the facial nerve are unable to close their eye tightly

A____ B____ C____ D____ E____

25. The external jugular vein:
(A) forms by union of the posterior auricular vein and the posterior branch of the retromandibular vein in the neck
(B) is subcutaneous on the surface of the sternocleidomastoid
(C) receives the facial vein
(D) drains into the subclavian vein
(E) drains into the internal jugular vein

A____ B____ C____ D____ E____

Answers to Multiple Choice Questions

1. A T	B T	C T	D F	E F	10. A F	B T	C T	D F	E F	19. A T	B F	C T	D F	E T
2. A T	B F	C T	D F	E F	11. A F	B T	C T	D T	E F	20. A F	B F	C T	D T	E T
3. A F	B F	C T	D F	E T	12. A F	B T	C F	D F	E T	21. A F	B F	C F	D F	E T
4. A T	B T	C F	D F	E F	13. A F	B T	C F	D T	E F	22. A F	B T	C T	D F	E F
5. A T	B F	C F	D T	E F	14. A F	B T	C T	D T	E T	23. A T	B F	C T	D T	E T
6. A F	B F	C T	D T	E T	15. A T	B T	C T	D T	E T	24. A T	B T	C F	D T	E F
7. A F	B T	C F	D F	E T	16. A T	B T	C T	D T	E T	25. A T	B T	C F	D T	E F
8. A F	B F	C T	D T	E F	17. A F	B T	C T	D T	E F					
9. A T	B T	C F	D F	E F	18. A F	B T	C T	D F	E F					

Index

Numbers in *italics* refer to illustrations